OZZY'S GIRLS

THE STORY OF THE GUTSY WOMEN WHO BUILT A HEALTHCARE EMPIRE

TERRI WALLO STRAUSS

Ava~
I hope you enjoy
reading Ozzy's Girls!
Love,
Terri Wallo Strauss

ISBN 978-1-7376372-0-2-E-book
ISBN 978-1-7376372-1-9 Hardcover
ISBN 978-1-7376372-2-6 Paperback
One Punch Productions, LLC
Ozzysgirls.com

CONTENTS

ACKNOWLEDGEMENTS FROM THE AUTHOR

This book was years in the making, as I was fortunate enough to grow up surrounded by some of Ozzy's Girls (a self-proclaimed term). In later years, I attended their annual Homecoming, where they gathered to share stories and their unbreakable bond. I also spent hours interviewing my mom, Dee Rennie Wallo. She would laugh at me for even thinking her story could be a book, but was still happy to launch into a tale about her training and the hospital. Much of the words in this book are her words, either told to me or written in the *Vincenette*, the biannual newsletter she wrote for the St. Vincent Nurses Alumnae.

In capturing the history of Ozzy's Girls as well as Providence St. Vincent Medical Center, I was able to rely on mountains of memorabilia; when one of Ozzy's Girls would pass, their families would give boxes of material to my mom, who had become the default archivist. Thank you to those families, for these gifts made this possible. Thank you to the unnamed person from the Class of 1954 who kept a detailed scrapbook that rivaled the National Archives—filled with brochures, news articles, photos and more. It was invaluable.

I wish I could have told all the stories and featured all the photos of every graduate, but alas, this is only one book.

Thank you to all those who consented to interviews or supplied even more information, including Chuck Blickle, Helen Clark, Mary Raglione Liefeld, Lynne Zuelke Magner, Rose Scherzinger, Susie Zuelke, and Pat Van Loo. Thank you to Peter Schmid, Providence Archives, for your efficiency and assistance with photos.

Special love and thanks to my mom's great friend, Dorothy Kennedy, and her daughters, Lori and Susan. Dorothy, thank you not only for being there for our mother, but for mothering me now. Lori, thank you for always making us laugh during Homecoming setup; watching Ozzy's Girls gather was always a highlight. And Susan, thank you for finding all the photos I kept asking for.

Thank you to my sister, MaryJo McCloskey, for her constant encouragement, sending me positive messages telling me I could do this. Thank you to my brothers, Edward and Steve Wallo, for supporting me and for trusting me to tell our mother's story.

To my husband, Scott, and my daughters, Delanie, Genna and Cara, thank you for putting up with my insecurities, especially when I asked if anyone would care about this story besides me. Thank you to my stepdaughter, Marisa, for your constant enthusiasm over this project. And to all my friends who listened endlessly about the need to tell this story—thank you. You know who you are.

Thank you to my editors, Suzanne Eggleston and Cindy Wallo, for agreeing to work on this project. I relied on your wisdom and ruthlessness. Thank you, Marshall Santos for your gifted graphics work.

This story is two-fold. First, it was important to capture the spirit of our mom, Dee Rennie Wallo, for future generations. There are great-grandchildren who will never know her and feel the warmth of her amazing smile. The second reason became so apparent in writing this: it was time to tell the story of these fearless, hardworking and gutsy women who braved such turbulent times while being at the forefront of a dizzying number of medical advancements.

From the beginning of the Sisters of Providence to Ozzy herself and her students, this story is about the power of strong women.

Here's to Ozzy's Girls.

Update:

When I started writing this book, it was years before the COVID-19 global pandemic. I never expected the toll this would take on our world, especially the healthcare system. In addition to Ozzy's Girls, I dedicate this book to the selfless and dedicated healthcare workers who are true heroes in this pandemic. They are on the front lines of crisis unlike anything our country has seen for a century. We will never forget their sacrifices.

Ozzy's Girls would be proud.

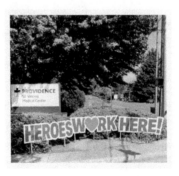

For Mom

PROLOGUE

Terri woke up with a start—disoriented as to what woke her. She soon realized it was the incessant ringing of her phone. Fumbling for it in the dark, she squinted and saw the number: It was her 81-year-old mother calling. Nothing good can come from a phone call at 3 a.m., Terri thought.

"Mom, what's the matter?" Terri asked, skipping the preliminaries and sounding calmer than she felt.

"I'm having an asthma attack," her mother gasped.

"Do I need to call an ambulance?" Terri asked, already getting out of bed, silently marveling again at her composure.

"No. Just get here," her mother said with emphasis.

Terri dove into clothes as if she was a seasoned first responder. The roughly three-mile drive to her mother's house never seemed so long, but she made good use of time, calling her sister and telling her to meet them at the hospital. Terri drove by Providence St. Vincent Medical Center on her way, glancing quickly at it, almost as if she was trying to assess if they were ready for an incoming patient.

Once at her mom's house, Terri let herself in and ran toward her mom's bedroom at the back of the house. Her eyes quickly darted around the bedroom, taking in her mom, who was sitting on the bed, gasping for air. A medical book and a blood pressure cuff lay next to her. Terri silently wondered how long her mom had debated about calling for help.

Despite the time it took to bundle her mom into her robe, climb under the dresser to find her slippers and grab her wallet, Terri was able to usher her mom into the car in minutes. Terri drove back to the hospital, mostly in silence, save for her mom's frequent gasps for air.

"It's going to be fine, Mom," Terri said, trying to sound reassuring. Turning quickly into the driveway of the Emergency Department, she drove straight up to the door under the portico. Without a word, her mom jumped out of the car, almost before it stopped. Though she didn't like her mom going in by herself, Terri realized that this could speed up the check-in process and her mom might be seen by a doctor sooner.

After parking nearby, Terri climbed out of her car and sprinted through the doorway. She glanced to her left and noticed a woman holding a small child. The woman gave Terri a stricken look, which puzzled her until she looked to her right.

"Mom!" Terri screamed, running over to the Emergency Department lobby floor, where her mom was now lying face down. Dropping to her knees, Terri touched her mom's coat. She looked down at the blood on her own hands quizzically until she saw the pool of blood that was seeping out near her mom's head.

"Oh God, Mom," Terri cried. Her mom must have been too weak and fell, Terri thought, mentally berating herself for letting her mom walk in by herself.

"Rapid Response Team to the ED," a voice wailed over the loudspeaker. Terri watched in disbelief as nurses and

doctors emerged suddenly and came to examine her unconscious mother. Turning her over gently, they removed her
broken glasses and made plans to secure her neck, lift her,
and place her on a stretcher. They then rushed her through
the twin electronic doors. Terri ran behind them, still in
shock.

The medical team guided the stretcher into the room,
their movements well-coordinated. A balding older doctor,
small glasses perched on his head, came running in. He
issued orders to the staff who were grabbing supplies and
medications in response. Everyone was working calmly and
efficiently; this was obviously not their first code. The
doctor tried to intubate Terri's mom so she could get
oxygen. Holding the tube just outside her throat, the doctor
yelled there was too much blood in her airway. Terri
watched as they suctioned blood from her mom's throat and
quickly administered drugs through an IV they had hastily
put in. Terri and her mom had watched this procedure a
million times on one of their favorite medical shows; this
time it was real. Terri then noticed the heart monitor and
her own heart sank at the flat line that was running across
its screen.

With her back against a wall, Terri felt her knees giving
out and slid down, feeling faint. Less than an hour ago, she
was asleep and peaceful, having gone to bed content. Now,
she was living in a nightmare. She urged herself silently to
wake up so she could realize this was just a nightmare.

Suddenly, a voice out of the haze said urgently, "Dr. Sharff,
we have a pulse." Things began settling down, thanks to the
drugs and breathing tube. The monitor showed a heart
rhythm and Terri's own heart began to beat faster.

A nurse gently approached Terri, his Irish brogue a
soothing contrast to her distress. He used a warm washcloth
to wipe the blood from her hands. Terri blinked at him, not

really taking in what he was saying, but she physically began to relax, feeling a sense of comfort in his touch.

A gentle calm seemed to take over the room. Nurses came in and out, silently cleaning up the area, getting rid of used wrappers and medications and double-checking the IV.

Dr. Sharff sat down on the edge of a stool by his patient's head. With his glasses on, he moved the overhead lamp and quietly stitched up the cut on the patient's forehead, which had taken the brunt of her fall. As he stood, he removed the blue suture paper cloth that had been covering most of his patient's head. Dr. Sharff's eyes suddenly widened. For the first time, he appeared almost excited.

"Oh my God, this is Dee Wallo"! Dr. Sharff exclaimed, glancing around at the nurses. "Hi Dee"! he said, nonsensically waving at her, although she was unconscious. The others looked at each other and then back at him questioningly.

"It's Dee Wallo!" he repeated, as if he was trying to make himself understood. "She used to run this place!"

SERVING OTHERS CHARTS THE COURSE

For as long as she could remember, Rose Marie "Dee" Rennie wanted to be a nurse. There would be no wavering in her decision, and no deterring her by others. She joked later in life that it was because she looked so good in white, a startling contrast with her olive skin and jet-black hair. No one knows why there was such a strong desire, but maybe because Dee's family life had centered on taking care of others, she was decisive about her profession. Her parents and those around her had a spirit of generosity and the desire to serve—something required of a nurse. Their lives had been built on strength and perseverance, and Dee reflected that. She was steadfast in her decision and maintained the stubbornness she so often displayed when she was passionate about something.

Dee's parents, Frank and Theresa Rennie, met in 1920, shortly after Frank had crossed over the border from Canada. Frank and his cousin Pete were young, strapping Sicilians, in their early 20s, on the short, stout side, with full heads of black, curly hair. The Rennie gene was a strong one, and they looked remarkably alike, sometimes getting confused by people who knew them well. Young Francesco's (his birth name) family and extended family had traveled to Winnipeg, Canada, from the mountainous region of Caccamo, Sicily. For reasons never discussed, the original family name of Rini was largely left behind in Sicily.

More family settled in Winnipeg over the years, and Frank and Pete grew up surrounded by multiple siblings and cousins. They spent their days skipping school to play ice hockey, their heads full of potential escapades. It was that sense of adventure and the longing to have a better life that led them to hatch a plan to travel to America when they reached adulthood. Learning that the small city of Portland, Oregon, possibly had jobs in the shipyard, they embarked with a small amount of money in their pockets and dreams in their heads.

Once in Portland, the two young Rennie cousins surveyed their situation. Portland was still a sleepy town compared to Seattle to the north and San Francisco to the south—both cities were far more cosmopolitan. Portland's downtown was growing, but immigrants clustered in specific neighborhoods around the city. With the Columbia River to the north and the Willamette River creating a natural east-west divider, Portland and its shipyards drew many men—including the young cousins—with the promise of employment.

Their paths took a different direction, however, when they met other Italians who were produce men and made their living selling fruits and vegetables. Being entrepreneurs held a certain allure, and despite a lack of much formal education, the cousins dove in headfirst, working harder than ever to get their business off the ground. They made a great team: Frank was wickedly smart and could do sums in his head faster than any modern calculator. He was big-hearted but somewhat introspective, confident in his dream of a vast enterprise. Of the two, Pete was the extrovert. A true salesperson, he would talk to anyone he came across, dance all night until the sun rose, and turn on the charm at will. The cousins were well-liked by others in the produce world, and they quickly started building their business from a small stand on Southeast Grand Avenue—known informally in town as "The Market."

The cousins soon made friends who lived in Ladd's Addition, a neighborhood in Southeast Portland that boasted large Craftsman-style homes, majestic elm trees, and narrow streets with alleyways. The area in Portland was once owned by merchant William S. Ladd, who developed the land before becoming Portland's mayor. Ladd was apparently inspired by Pierre Charles L'Enfant's plans for Washington, D.C. Ladd imagined this new neighborhood shaped as a diagonal wagon-wheel arrangement, with four diamond-shaped rose gardens. A central roundabout surrounding a park was the area's landmark.

Multitudes of Italian families had settled in Ladd's Addition over the years, while other Italians in the city had settled on the west side of town. Westside Italians became forever known as the "ones with money." Eastside Italians were known to be scrappier, making do with little, but united in the American way to build a fresh start and prosper.

One day, the Rennie cousins walked into a small corner store in Ladd's Addition and ran smack into the Greco girls. The two sisters were manning the small family run "store"—a term far grander than the real thing. The tiny kiosk was filled with a few staples their neighbors might need, such as flour and sugar. Neither sister could have known that the incoming men were to become their future husbands.

Theresa Greco and her sister, Salvadora, known as Dorothy outside the family, were just under two years apart in age, and as close as any sisters could be. They both had black eyes and straight black hair, which they stubbornly tried to curl. Although alike in appearance, they were very different in character. Theresa, the older sister (then 19), was petite, had an iron will, spoke her mind freely and traveled with confidence. Dorothy, or "Dode" as Theresa lovingly called her, was on the plump side. She was a hard worker, had an infectious laugh and a forgiving nature.

The sisters came from a family who had made their life in Portland in the late 1800s. Their father, Antonio, had traveled to San Francisco from their small fishing village of Trabia, Sicily. Five years later, Antonio had earned enough money to send for his bride, Prudentia, their three children, and his mother-in-law. They soon traveled to Portland after hearing there were more jobs up north.

Antonio and Prudentia settled in, having four more children, including Theresa and Dorothy, with one son unfortunately dying at the age of 12. They raised their six children in this unique neighborhood that centered around St. Philip Neri Catholic Church, where Paulist priests had eventually gathered enough money to buy land for a small church. In fact, this effort was undertaken by Antonio and the parish priest, who traveled by horse and buggy each Sunday to go door-to-door asking for donations. Never mind that the two were on a Catholic fundraising mission, they came home each week tipsy, shrugging it off and explaining that a drink of homemade wine at each house was only being *polite*.

Having been born in Portland at the turn of the century, Theresa and Dorothy told everyone they were American. They embraced their new heritage, loving high fashion, speaking English outside of the home and championing women's rights, even at their young age. Their favorite hobby was to dress up and have glamor shots taken, clad in their best dresses, their large hats sitting delicately on their carefully curled hair, their muskrat throws around their necks.

The girls had both reluctantly left high school to work

and help the family weather the years during World War I. As the older of the two sisters, Theresa was intended to marry first. As she and Frank began to court; however, it was soon apparent he was focused on building his business before anything. Methodical in nature, he took his time.

So, it was with a little guilt, but the yearning of true young love, that Dorothy and Pete quietly eloped with no family present. Theresa understood and never held it against Dorothy. After Theresa and Frank married in 1922 and rented a home on Southeast 20th and Clinton, the sisters—and cousins—were together again when Dorothy and Pete moved in right next door.

And since they did everything together, Dorothy and Theresa also found themselves pregnant at the same time. Theresa gave birth to a daughter during Labor Day weekend in 1924. She was to be an only child, and the photos of her reflect her parents' unwavering attention. Dressed in fine garments, often with delicate jewelry, their baby already had a big smile and a little head of black curls. Italian tradition necessitated that she be named after Frank's mother, Rosaria. Unfortunately, Theresa didn't get on fabulously with her very forceful mother-in-law, who Frank had now settled in the Portland area with his father and four siblings. Theresa grimaced at the thought; she instead championed the name Marie. The couple finally was forced to compromise and named their daughter Rose Marie. As with most compromises, neither was entirely happy with the name. For a couple years, Theresa rebelliously just called her new daughter "Baby."

Fate soon intervened. Dorothy had given birth to a boy and named him John Frederick. As a toddler, John attempted to say Rose Marie, but in his simple language skills, it came out sounding like "Dee Dee." That suited everyone just fine. From then on, the relieved family only called little Rose

Marie, "Dee." Dee was also finding it challenging to pronounce John Frederick, and proclaimed him "Fef." That stuck as well, at least inside the family.

Unfortunately, Dee was a sickly child. She contracted a severe infection when she was a toddler—the infection nearly took her life and left her at risk for every other ear infection or virus that came along. She even had an emergency tracheotomy before it was even attempted by most local doctors.

Theresa was understandably frightened and did what any self-respecting mother would do, especially one surrounded by decades of Italian tradition: She took Dee to a healer. Old Mrs. Fracasso laid hands on Dee, but it didn't take. Dee got what was thought to be rheumatic fever around age 11, and it hit her hard. She recovered, but the doctor told her worried parents it also left Dee with a damaged heart valve. Best not to tax her heart, the doctor cautioned. "No exercise, no work, no having children. She will have to take life easy," he said.

In the community of Ladd's Addition, everyone knew everyone, and a kid couldn't walk three houses without a full report by the "Mother Squad." Therefore, Dee spent her days feeling a little trapped, sitting on the wide porch stairs of the family's home, watching the neighbor kids running and playing ball. She was forbidden from learning to swim, ride a bicycle or run. She yearned to be treated the same as every other kid.

The closest Dee came to that normalcy she craved was when she spent time with the only non-Italian family in the neighborhood. Her close friend Norma Thompson and her parents were big strapping people of Swedish descent. They all loved the outdoors. Norma, blonde, robustly healthy and almost a head taller, was a remarkable contrast to the petite, dark Dee.

The Thompsons insisted on taking Dee with them to the

Oregon Coast, which was about 75 miles away. The family would stay down there after the long drive and enjoy the coast, watching in awe as the powerful Pacific Ocean crashed against the rugged shore. Dee loved the Oregon Coast, and these trips meant everything to her, providing a sense of normalcy as she dug for clams and ran on the sand.

As Dee grew, Frank and his cousin, Pete, continued growing their business as well, despite the Depression. They began to travel to California to pick up fresh fruits and vegetables, employing a couple of nephews on the side.

Meanwhile, Theresa had gone to work at a bank after convincing a neighbor to teach her how to drive. Frank wasn't against her driving; in fact, he championed it. However, he valued his life more, and with great trepidation he watched his 4-foot-9 wife drive away, her tiny head barely above the dashboard of the large car. He seemed to understand that he married an independent woman who did not want to stay at home in a traditional role; the two forged ahead with plans for their future with her working outside the home. Theresa became the neighborhood's de facto driver, often shuttling her friends to the store or the doctor, happy to be independent. She loved to be out of the house, often saying "there is no future in housework." Dorothy would laugh, quietly, going about her chores as well as Theresa's, cooking and sewing for both families.

Life took a horrific turn in 1933 when Frank received a frantic call from his nephew, relaying that Pete had succumbed likely to a heart attack. The two were on their way home from California, when Pete died beside the truck, just outside the city of Roseburg, roughly four hours south of Portland. He was just 37 years old. Frank locked himself in the bathroom, overcome with grief, and could not go next door to tell Dorothy that she was now a single mother of four. Theresa, always the stronger one of the couple, bore the news to her sister, who was busy preening in a mirror, trying on a new red dress because she and Pete had planned to go dancing upon his return.

Frank moved his cousin's family in with them for a while. Dee's four cousins, already close, became almost her siblings. Dee's best friend was Fef. Quiet and steady, he was often by her side, always protective. His brother Anthony or "Nini," had a sizeable piece of her heart as well. Shorter and stout with a wide smile, Nini had a great sense of humor and his dad's dancing gene. Just a year younger than Dee and Fef, Nini was used to lagging behind the pair. He made up for it on the dance floor, flinging Dee around, laughing all the way. Rounding out the trio of boys was Eugene. Slighter and quieter than the other two, he developed polio as a child, walking with a slight limp. The baby of the cousins was Marge: younger than the rest, gregarious and fun, she routinely ran off with other girls in the neighborhood on one adventure or another.

Meanwhile, Frank continued to build his business, now in the shadow of his best friend's and cousin's death. Working with a few nephews, he got the idea to buy a refrigerated truck that ran on butane, virtually unheard of in those days. He could keep the produce fresher during the long hauls, Frank thought, already planning his fortune. However, on a trip back from Los Angeles, the kindhearted Frank picked up a hitchhiker who lit a cigarette, causing the truck to burn beyond repair.

The incident almost ruined Frank financially, but he bounced back yet again. Frank borrowed some money and bought a new truck. Now a confident businessperson, he met a man from Armenia named Charlie Mohawkian. They formed M&R Produce and started making money through the government. They rattled down the old highway west to the Oregon Coast, bringing produce to the government-spon-

sored work camps, where men were busy with forest manage-
ment as well as building roads and tunnels and other
infrastructure. This work was part of then President Franklin
D. Roosevelt's New Deal, which included the Civilian
Conservation Corps. It was a highly profitable venture for
small businesses, but Frank's trips took days and were long
and arduous.

With his good fortune, however, Frank could finally buy a
home in Ladd's Addition on 21st Avenue and Cyprus Street
for Theresa, Dee and the family dog, Micky. Dorothy and her
family moved nearby. Things were improving and Frank
employed several nephews and loaned money to those who
needed it—always too kind to say no. A dapper dresser, he
got the nickname "Uncle Sheiky" from his nephews, referring
to the popular 1920s' film, *The Sheik*.

Frank and Theresa were generous with extended family,
especially when bad fortune hit again. Theresa's brother, Joe,
suffered the loss of his wife. A man raising an adolescent
daughter was unheard of in those days, so Joe dropped off his
teenage daughter, Theresa, known as Trixie. Although Trixie
and Dee were a few years apart, the two shared a room and a
small bond. Tragedy continued to strike, though, when Trixie
was killed in a car crash with her boyfriend. She was only 19.

Despite all the adversity, the family persisted, working
hard, but always with a lot of laughter. Now even more
cousins from both sides of the family had moved in just
blocks away. The relatives came over for Sunday dinners—the
big table always filled with spaghetti, meatballs and ended
with cheese and nuts. Wine was made in great big barrels in
the basement, as it had been for most of Prohibition in years
prior. The house's faded floral wallpaper soaked up the laughter. Dee, an only child, was never alone.

Dee went to nearby Abernethy Grade School with many
of her cousins. When the teacher said the name Rennie,

more than one hand shot in the air. It was difficult when Dee graduated and began attending nearby Washington High School, as it forced her to be separated from Fef, who was sent to a local boys' preparatory school, Benson Tech High School. Fef was always sensitive to Dee's feelings, so he walked the extra miles to "pick her up" and walk her home each day.

Dee earned good grades and reportedly only got called to the principal's office once. Dee's offense was allegedly assaulting her lab partner. Theresa drove her big car down to pick up Dee, and without even blinking an eye, dressed the principal down for making a big deal out of nothing. On the way home, Dee tried to explain she just got angry that her lab partner failed to do her share of the work. Dee claimed all she did was grab the girl by the arms to make her point. "Listen here," Dee said to the girl, "You haven't done a thing and I'm doing all the work!" Theresa, just drove on, silently listening to Dee, trusting her daughter's account, secretly proud that she was raising a confident and strong daughter.

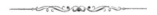

No one saw it coming—at least in their tiny part of the world. When Pearl Harbor was attacked in 1941, those in Portland felt immediately threatened. The Pacific Northwest wasn't that far from Hawaii, they thought with panic. If the country was now at war and Hawaii had been a target, what was to keep the enemy from using the Pacific Ocean to come ashore at the Oregon Coast?

When the news of Pearl Harbor hit, Frank was driving up from California, his truck loaded with produce. Theresa knew in her heart that he was fine, but she couldn't convince her 17-year-old daughter of that. She did everything she could to settle Dee's mind, finally dragging her to a movie, a true luxury in those days. Dee was distraught, fearing the worst, sick at the thought that her kind, hardworking dad would be in harm's way. She never remembered what movie she saw.

When Frank arrived home safely, Dee was greatly relieved, but the family continued to live in fear. Others in their small community did as well, glued to their radios each night for news of the war. Climbing under their desks became a mandatory and frequent bombing drill in Dee's high school classes.

Dee watched with great sadness as her schoolmates of Japanese descent disappeared one by one from her high school, most interned with their families at camps in Eastern Oregon and other rural spots. The unfairness of it all upset Dee, but she realized the fear permeating society was misdirected toward those of Japanese descent—many of whom were American citizens.

The fear kept growing with each news report and the neighbors in Ladd's Addition cobbled together a citizen militia, a roughshod group of Italian men who dusted off their old pheasant hunting rifles. They decided they would begin training to shoot the enemy if they landed on American shores and made their way to Portland.

For most people, life suddenly had turned upside down. Dee watched with a heavy heart as most of her male cousins enlisted in the armed services and left their safe neighborhood one by one. They were 17, 18, 19 and beyond, and they were now slipping away from her. Life once so simple was now far more complex. Dee watched as Fef, and later Nini, joined the Army and shipped out. Their younger brother, Eugene, was not accepted because of his medical complications. Even Theresa's brother, Tony, who was now in his late 30s, was drafted to drive a truck in the Army. Married to Frank's sister Lena, the couple had no children of their own and had been a constant in Dee's life. Dee watched her uncle and aunt drive off, headed to the South, away from any family. Lena leaned out the window, waving frantically to Dee, her brown eyes misting behind her cat-eye glasses, until the car turned the corner, leaving Ladd's Addition.

Meanwhile, Dee graduated from high school and was happy to finish. Her yearbook speaks to her desire for continuing her education, listing her as "college prep." The yearbook editors also took license to find one sentence to describe her adequately: "One who is always full of glee, is our dark and pretty Dee."

Dee grew up surrounded by love, hard work, some sadness, compromise and most of all, the spirit of generosity. It was all this, plus her own illnesses, that ingrained in her a willingness to serve as a nurse. There was to be no compromise when she declared her wish to attend the St. Vincent School of Nursing.

NUNS OF STEEL

It is said that greatness can be achieved by standing on the shoulders of those who have come before you. Dee did not know yet about the greatness achieved by the Sisters of Providence—but she would come to learn and value their sacrifices.

In all started in 1800, in a small house near the center of Montreal, Canada, when Emilie Tavernier Gamelin was born, the youngest of 15 children. Unfortunately, only six would survive.

Even as a small child, Emilie was generous and enthusiastically gathered food items in sacks to give to those who were financially struggling in Montreal. Emilie's life was not to be easy, though. Her mother died when she was just four years old. Her father and sister followed in death; fortunately, an aunt adopted Emilie. When Emilie was 18, she went to live with her brother after he lost his wife, and took charge of his household. Her brother graciously granted Emilie her wish to use the dining room as a headquarters for her charities.

When Emilie was 23, she married Jean Baptiste, who at 50 was very much her senior. A prominent Montreal citizen, he agreeably shared his wealth and allowed Emilie to continue with her charity work.

Emilie's life continued in sorrow as two of the couple's three children died as young toddlers. Later, her husband died as well as her one surviving son.

These final blows were just about all Emilie could take, and she soon found the only escape from her grief was through helping others. She continued her work through the Ladies of Charity of Montreal, reaching out to the elderly and those imprisoned or suffering from afflictions, mental illness and disabilities.

Emilie had no idea that she was about to face even more tragedy. In 1833, a ship traveling from an Irish port landed in Quebec. When the 133 passengers disembarked, it was discovered 59 people had died at sea. In the following six days, there were 216 additional deaths. It was soon learned the plague had come to Canada. Despite the danger, Emilie cared for these cholera victims, including the new orphans and widows. She soon became known as the Mother of the Poor. People she helped said it was providence that brought her to them.

Emilie's renowned reputation soon gained the attention of Bishop Ignace Bourget of Montreal. He created a charitable community in 1843, with Emilie becoming the first Mother Superior. Her reign was just eight years, as she died of cholera in 1851. Her last words to her fellow sisters were "humility, simplicity, charity." With that direction, Emilie had left a tremendous legacy: The Sisters of Charity of Providence, Servants of the Poor, who went by the name of the Sisters of Providence for practical reasons.

Whatever the name, the Sisters of Providence were a force to be reckoned with. A small troop of these Catholic Sisters, led by Mother Joseph of the Sacred Heart, who had worked alongside Emilie, traveled from Montreal to Vancouver, Washington, to start a mission to serve the sick and poor.

One has to have empathy for the four sisters who accompanied Mother Joseph—she probably kept them soldiering on no matter what adversity was in their tracks.

The daughter of a Montreal carriage-maker, architect and artisan in wood, Mother Joseph had learned a lot along the way. She was remarkably a builder, architect, carpenter, engineer, artist, woodcarver and general handyperson. In fact, when a young Mother Joseph, then known as Esther Pariseau, was presented by her father to Mother Emilie, he spoke proudly of the skills he had instilled in his daughter: "She [Esther] has learned carpentry from me and can handle tools as well as I can. Moreover, she can plan and supervise the work of others. I assure you, Madame, she will someday make a very good [Mother] Superior."

Mother Emilie took her on and the two were a powerful team. Now, with Mother Emilie gone, Mother Joseph carried Emilie's strength and spirit, and led her fellow sisters with confidence. Petite with beady eyes, a large nose and straight mouth, Mother Joseph was far more imposing than her stature.

Once the sisters arrived in Vancouver, they first built Providence Academy, a day school and orphanage. After additional reinforcement sisters arrived, the group concentrated on building a small hospital.

Mother Joseph's work did not go unnoticed. As the nearby city of Portland, Oregon, grew with a population of about 9,000, F.N. Blanchet, bishop of the Diocese of Oregon City, sent word for the Sisters of Providence to cross the Columbia River and start a new hospital. Mother Joseph, a woman of action, readily agreed to at least discuss it.

A decade went by as the sisters prayed and tried to figure out how to finance the building of a hospital in Portland. In fact, the nuns had become quite good at the fundraising business, using unique methods to garner cash. In the mid-1860s,

Mother Joseph had an interesting idea. Why not go directly to local goldminers and catch them at the very source of their discoveries before they had a chance to travel to nearby towns and cities to spend their fortunes? To fund their various missions and philanthropic ventures, the sisters fanned out and headed in various directions.

Realizing one of her character flaws was the lack of a warm personality, Mother Joseph carefully chose her traveling companion. Sister Catherine, a quick-witted, genteel Irish woman, was the perfect sidekick. The two ventured east to Idaho, where they climbed down mine shafts to confront wary miners. The sisters faced rough horseback rides, wolves, forest fires and even potential robbers; the sometimes arrogant and hostile miners were not even a challenge.

Sadly, they still didn't have the funds to build the hospital in Portland, but it became more feasible when in 1874, the local St. Vincent de Paul Society was able to raise $1,000 and a gift of land in Northwest Portland. Mother Joseph opened a letter that informed her about the land donation on July 19, which was then the Feast Day of St. Vincent de Paul (it was later changed to September 27 following the reform of the General Roman Calendar). Mother Joseph believed it was a sign that the new hospital should be named for the patron saint of taking care of those in need. She immediately began designing St. Vincent Hospital.

Meanwhile, across the country, another Sister of Providence, Mother Mary Theresa, was quietly running a hospital and orphanage in Burlington, Vermont. In her late 30s, Mother Mary Theresa was described as a person of rare strength and individualism. When she got word about the need in Portland, Mother Mary Theresa, a committed healer, got on a train—and later a ship—to travel up the mighty Columbia River to rendezvous with her fellow sisters in Vancouver, Washington.

The sisters continued fundraising in Portland, even going door to door, asking residents for spare cash for the new hospital. This effort was difficult, given the French-speaking sisters' broken English, and an overall dislike of Catholics in the city (Portlanders were predominantly Protestant at this time). The sisters persevered, though, and were able to raise more than $1,600. A public bazaar raised another $2,500. With less than $5,000 in their pockets, construction started on a hospital in what is now Portland's renowned Pearl District which features shops, upscale townhomes and trendy restaurants. In the late 1800s, however, it was a sparsely populated industrial section of town bordering Couch Lake (which was later filled in to build Union Station).

Mother Joseph's design and construction skills, combined with Mother Mary Theresa's knowledge in administration and finance, made them the medical facility dream team of the 1800s. The very next day, the sisters adopted a plan drafted by Mother Joseph. Construction began, but the workers had no idea what they were getting into with their new contractor. Mother Joseph, her black habit with the white wimple surrounding her face, and giant skirts blowing in the wind, was said to be seen bouncing on a high cross-beam to test its strength or ripping up flooring to see what was underneath.

Oregon historian and author Ellis Lucia chronicled the building of the hospital in his 1975 book, *Cornerstone*. Later, he relayed to *The Oregonian* newspaper a particular story:

"Once when overseeing the project, Mother Joseph ordered a brick chimney constructed from a solid base on the ground. That evening when making her inspection of the day's work, she found to her disgust that the masons had set the chimney base on the flooring. Muttering some brief prayer, which was her style as she moved about, Mother Joseph rolled up her sleeves and the bricks came tumbling down. The next morning when the workmen returned, they found the chimney had been completely re-laid, but this time firmly on the ground."

As the building grew closer to reality, the nuns had to retreat to Vancouver for the tough winter—much to the relief of the construction crew. When they returned hoping to find their shiny new hospital, the sisters were in for a significant disappointment: The hospital was in disarray. Clutter was everywhere, including pieces of lumber, unfinished plaster, paint, dirt and dust. Prayers were undoubtedly uttered again, but the nuns rolled up their sleeves while they did it. Mother Mary Theresa bought cleaning materials on credit, and the nuns performed back-breaking labor to get the 16,000-square-foot building presentable.

Though the formal dedication of the hospital was scheduled for July, the first patients began arriving prior to that, and Mother Mary Theresa, acting as the hospital's first administrator, welcomed them. Their first patient was George Allen, a 22-year-old plumber who arrived on their doorstep on June 24. Dr. Alfred Kinney, an Oregon native, had attended Bellevue Hospital Medical School in New York, but agreed to travel back to Portland to be the hospital's first doctor. He wrote about the unofficial opening years later in a letter to his nephew:

"The first patient was a wounded Scandinavian [Allen], brought up by boat from Oak Point. I took him from the steamboat in my buggy to the hospital and carried him (170 lbs.) up the long steps, through the front door and onto the operating room where I,

with blessed Sister Peter Claver administering chloro-
form, fixed him up."

This first patient was desperately ill, and was said to have
"a wicked life," but the sisters were able to nurse him back to
health. He later stayed on to work for $1.50 a week to pay off
part of his hospital bill.

The next few patients, also non-Catholics, were taken
care of as well, and the sisters silently sent up a prayer, hoping
this would quell any notion that their hospital was for
Catholics only. Their three-story, wood-framed, 75-bed
hospital was located on what is now Northwest 12th between
Marshall and Northrup, and came in at just over $22,000 in
construction costs.

Dedication day for Oregon's first permanent hospital was on
July 19, of course, in 1875. Mother Joseph even carved a statue of
St. Vincent de Paul, which stood proudly on the hospital roof.
On this beautiful day in July, thousands crowded the streets to
watch the ceremonies orchestrated by the St. Vincent de Paul
Society. At 2 p.m., the band began playing and a procession of
men in uniforms representing various associations and organi-
zations began marching proudly from downtown to the new
hospital. The newspapers reported on this large celebration, yet
there was no mention in the speeches or newspaper of Mother
Joseph or Mother Mary Theresa, their vision or their hard work.

There was no downtime for the sisters, however. After the
ceremony, at 8 p.m., a horse-drawn ambulance brought a critical patient, a man named Joe, whose arm was badly injured
and needed amputation. The man eventually recovered and
paid for his care in full: $21 for 21 days in the hospital.

The hospital came at a time when the average life span
for a man was 47 years old, and patients paid $1 a day for
treatment (paid either in cash, by barter, or written off as

charity). Medications were extra and included bourbon, an all-purpose pain reliever also known as a cure for "snakebite" —a legend from the Oregon frontier.

In the first year, the sisters admitted 320 patients, of which 285 were discharged and 30 died. The sisters treated everyone—from those injured by gunshots to typhoid or toothaches. Others had heart disease, torpidity of the bowels, malaria, syphilis and more. More men than woman were patients and often, they stayed a month or more wanting free food and board.

The sisters, ever generous, continued to take care of any charity patients who came their way, buying what they needed on credit. Their mortgage holders got nervous, and the nuns knew it was time to extend their fundraising efforts.

Sister Joseph of Arimathea and Sister Perpetua modeled their own begging tour after Mother Joseph's earlier mine fundraising. They traveled through the Willamette Valley, but didn't find much. It wasn't until they arrived in Coos Bay and North Bend that they met with some success. A local paper published a story about the new hospital and said St. Vincent was a place "where all are admitted whatever their color, nationality or religion." This gave the sisters and the hospital greater credibility and donations came in at a steadier, but slower pace. "Beginnings are always trying," Mother Joseph wrote to the Mother House in Montreal.

When they weren't fundraising, Mother Mary Theresa and her small band of sisters not only acted as nurses, but were also in charge of cleaning, washing, food service and record keeping. Mother Mary Theresa urged the sisters to read medical books in the hospital's growing library, including one called the *Little Medical Guide of the Sisters of Charity of Providence,* continually updated by the Mother House. They went to lectures by the hospital's new doctors and were taught how to apply bandages, make beds and other tasks. The sisters were able to add two more wings shortly thereafter, in 1880 and 1883, bringing patient capacity to 150.

Meanwhile, communicable diseases began to enter the hospital, including scarlet fever, typhoid and meningitis. The real fear came with the epidemic of smallpox, which the sisters knew had killed so many Native American tribes in the years prior. The city had an isolation sanitarium which went by the unfortunate name "the Pest House," where Portlanders could go to hopefully recover. However, the cemetery next door was not encouraging, with the result that the hospital saw more smallpox patients trying to circumvent the Pest House. That was not tolerated; when patients were diagnosed with smallpox at the hospital, they were promptly sent to the Pest House and their rooms scrubbed clean and disinfected. Mother Mary Theresa worried the hospital would have to be shuttered. She and her fellow sisters prayed fervently. Those prayers must have worked; no more smallpox cases came, and Mother Mary Theresa's fears were not realized.

Additional challenges rose for the sisters: noise, pollution (from wood-burning stoves) and the growth in factories in the surrounding area was crowding the already full hospital. Mother Mary Theresa knew a medical crisis was brewing. After five years of searching and discussing the situation with Mother Joseph, Mother Mary Theresa discovered she needed only to look out her window to find the answer.

In 1888, Mother Mary Theresa decided the hospital's new home would be a mile west in the foothills of northwest Portland. The area was remote, sparsely populated, and full of trees, which meant it needed much excavation before building. Mother Mary Theresa began fundraising and eventually bought the five acres of land for $21,500, on what was then Cornell Street and later renamed Westover Road, despite the outcry from the doctors and even the sisters, who thought it was too far from downtown Portland.

The estimated cost of the new hospital was an ambitious $300,000. This amount was even more daunting when realizing the sisters would need to fundraise while also continuing to operate their current hospital. Mother Joseph once again bent over her drawing board, designing a modern Gibraltar-like structure, six stories high, and nestled close to the hill. Her plans would later be adapted by another architect, Justus F. Krumbein, as Mother Joseph went on to oversee other projects.

Each step of the way, the sisters struggled, and at one point borrowed more money. When the loan came due, a stubborn broker demanded payment in full. The sisters did the one thing that had never failed them before: pray. Those prayers were answered when the Sisters received an envelope of money from their Mother House.

Mother Mary Theresa was unaware that another crisis was literally at her doorstep. In 1894, floodwaters ascended more than 30 feet high—reaching the second story of the current hospital, and yet the sisters continued to care for their patients. Mother Mary Theresa was out of town on a trip to local missions. She had seen the headlines and anxiously had her travel partner send a telegram: "Has water reached the hospital? Mother Theresa much worried."

Mother Mary Theresa was right to be concerned. She arrived back at the hospital and was devastated to see the water's destruction and hear what her fellow sisters had gone through. She looked around at the industrial area that surrounded the hospital and wondered when the next flood would occur. She couldn't wait to get the new hospital built.

Mother Mary Theresa's dreams were finally realized almost 20 years to the day from the building of the first hospital. The new hospital accommodated 275 beds, and featured electric lighting instead of gas lighting, and wide corridors with high ceilings.

When it was officially dedicated in July 1895, the hospital was considered one of the country's premier medical facilities. The sisters watched the ceremony as men once again made speeches, though the sisters had spent several years gathering all the needed funds for construction and supervised its building. This time, it didn't go unnoticed.

In his book *Cornerstone*, Ellis Lucia summarized the speech by Dr. William Jones, who unknowingly gave the first plug in the state for the women's movement:

> "The hospital speaks eloquently of what women can accomplish in the conduct of large enterprises. Yet this great hospital was created, organized and is administered entirely by women. And the system of which it forms a part extending over the Northwest states and British Columbia is managed entirely by the Sisters of Providence. This is something for women to be proud of and speaks more highly of women's mental powers than all the successful books ever written by women."

One wonders if the sisters smiled at this overdue recognition. They must have certainly been proud of their accomplishment.

Located in what was then called Portland's "Crown of West Hills," the second St. Vincent Hospital had spacious operating rooms, elevators and hot water. The fee was $7 per week for a bed in a ward and $14 and up for private rooms. Each floor of the hospital consisted of three departments and was divided into sections based on the floor and geographic area it was located in (for example, 2 North). Some departments had bigger wards, with nine or even 15 beds at times.

There was not a bed #13 in the whole hospital—the nuns were superstitious that way.

Behind the hospital was a narrow alley where trucks could deliver goods to the hospital, and a small morgue. Over the years, footbridges were added, giving access quickly to the chapel, the interns' quarters and the sisters' convent.

In 1910, a south wing was added, a power plant soon after and later, an ice plant. Medicine was advancing quickly, and now the sisters had a modern facility to be at the forefront of it.

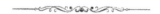

DURING THE BUILDING OF THIS MODERN HOSPITAL, THE sisters realized they needed more professional help in the way of nurses and opened a small nursing school. The first diploma from St. Vincent Training School was given to Rose Philpot in 1893. Rose was a laywoman who had been volunteering for the hospital since its opening.

The nuns then accelerated their efforts to train nurses. They opened a two- and later, a three-year nursing school, graduating another nurse, Agnes Johnston in 1894, after two years of training. The first full class of five students graduated in 1897. Rose Philpott was tapped to be an instructor. The sisters also hired Theresa Cox, who had trained at Bellevue Hospital in New York, and brought with her the first real textbook. The physicians were also the guest lecturers, and the students rotated through classes in departments such as obstetrics, surgery, dietary, public health, and others at St. Vincent Hospital. The classes each had about six to 10 graduates.

With the school showing promise, a new Nurses' Home for students to live in while training was built at the rear of the hospital in 1908. It sat as a tribute to Mother Mary

Theresa, who later died in 1921 at the age of 84, but not before seeing her hospital providing valued care for the community.

Through the years, the St. Vincent Training School's attendance increased. The decision was made to build another new Nurses' Home, a seven-story structure, to house the growing number of students attending the school. The new home was dedicated in 1931. The old Nurses' Home, St. Theresa Hall, up the hill and a little back from the hospital, was converted to classrooms.

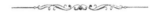

IT WAS JUST A FEW YEARS PRIOR THAT HARRIETT EDNA Osborn arrived in Oregon. Harriett hailed from the Yukon Territory in Canada and was looking forward to higher education. Growing up in the northern wilderness, with a father as a miner, Harriett had a rugged, outdoorsy nature. She decided to attend the University of Oregon and become a physical education teacher.

When Harriett arrived at the university, she discovered to her dismay that women were required to wear big bloomers and partake of sports in the sun. To be decked out in what she considered horrific long, billowing shorts in the bright sunlight (something she wasn't used to), was not an ideal situation.

If Harriett had liked suntans and bloomers, her tremendous influence on the next generation of nurses would never have occurred. Fortunately, she followed in her mother's footsteps to become a nurse.

In 1924, Harriett traveled up the hill to the University of Oregon Medical School (now the Oregon Health Sciences University) and then over to St. Vincent School of Nursing—a unique arrangement created by the St. Vincent School of

Nursing's dean, Sister Genevieve de Nanterre, RN, who was a 1914 graduate of the St. Vincent School of Nursing.

Sister Genevieve had come to the realization that nurses needed more training than their school could provide. She asked the university to assist, and Harriett was the first graduate with a Bachelor of Science in the five-year nursing course in 1929. The local newspaper, *The Oregonian*, wrote a story about "peculiar interest" surrounding the graduation of the first nurse in the State of Oregon to have a bachelor's degree. The next year, 44 nurses would follow in Harriett's footsteps.

Upon graduation, Harriett became the Director of Education for St. Vincent School of Nursing. She later said she simply had no choice, the nuns "grabbed her and thrust her into education," seeing firsthand the dedication Harriett had to developing the whole nurse through education and experience. Harriett overhauled the curriculum, grading system and instructors. Education was paramount in Harriett's mind, and she found like-minded thinking with Sister Genevieve. Sister Genevieve had already decided the hybrid education she had cobbled together was not a long-term solution, and the school needed more of a commitment from a higher learning institution. Sister Genevieve had approached Columbia University in Portland and asked for an affiliation so that graduates from the St. Vincent School of Nursing could receive a bachelor's degree.

Founded in 1901 as Columbia University and later renamed the University of Portland, the school sat back from rugged cliffs in North Portland and was aptly nicknamed "the Bluff." The university was operated by the Congregation of the Holy Cross—the same order of priests affiliated with the University of Notre Dame. At the time, the university consisted only of a few buildings and some land. Cash assets were said to be kept in three cigar boxes. Despite their meager resources, priests saw little need for expansion, as it was a men's institution until the School of Nursing came knocking.

Sister Genevieve was nothing if not tenacious. Negotiations between Sister Genevieve and the university's president, Rev. Joseph P. Boyle, finally ended with an agreement that ultimately got the nun what she wanted: nurses educated in a higher learning environment on their terms. The agreement said the university would act as an Extension Division and given free rein, allowing it to fix tuition, admission requirements, fees and other regulations. Approval of the superintendent of nurses at St. Vincent was still needed, however, to be accepted into the program. St. Vincent would still arrange for all clinical training.

In 1934, the 31 female students joining the all-male student body were met with some resistance. The university's student paper reported on the new agreement between the university and St. Vincent School of Nursing with the following article:

> "The ideals and traditions which have always been sacred to the stronger sex must now be shared with a group of young women who claim Columbia as their own."

The male student body soon relaxed when they realized the new female students wouldn't ever come on campus for academic reasons, and it would take four years before anyone even saw them at the graduation ceremonies. By that time, Columbia had transformed into the University of Portland.

The University of Portland embraced this partnership and advertised for nurses "of good health, sound character, an attractive personality, an interest in people and what interests people, and a willingness to work hard." They also appealed to those who "have a sincere desire to prepare for a career in

an important profession—nursing." The brochure was reassuring to those nursing candidates who were uncertain: "If,
after sincere effort, you find yourself miscast for the role of
nursing, leave with our best wishes."

The brochure was a sign of the times, and the priests
undoubtedly were sincere in their beliefs. They described the
importance of a Bachelor of Science degree:

- A college education
- More earning power
- Prestige
- Mental development
- Friendships

The power of nursing was described as meaning:

- Service to others
- A profession
- Security
- Unclaimed opportunities
- Preparation for marriage

And finally, the university boasted: "Probably the greatest
reward nurses receive for their work is the satisfaction of
having given service and happiness to mankind. No profession can claim greater reward. Nurses, because of their
training and experience, make splendid wives and mothers.
Monetary rewards are becoming increasingly satisfactory."

The marketing worked and the first graduating class in
1938 included 20 women who went to classes at St. Vincent,
trained at St. Vincent, and received bachelor's degrees from
the University of Portland. The University of Portland's yearbook, *The Log,* even carried a photo of the first graduating
class along with their activities and student council.

The school offered a four-year degree program and a five-year degree program for students who couldn't pay tuition and performed what is now commonly known as "work study." Tuition during this era ranged from $300, plus fees, for the first year; $180 for sophomores; $52.50 for juniors; and dwindling to just $30 for the final year. Despite the appeal for the nursing degree program, no one over the age of 30 was allowed, and it was offered only to single women.

Soon after the association with the University of Portland began, the federal government got involved in nursing. A federally funded Cadet Program was started to shore up the need for nurses. St. Vincent Hospital trained the cadets, who entered the three-year program. Cadets were also an invaluable factor in the school's ability to keep St. Vincent School of Nursing pumping out nurses even during the dark times of war.

The university should have created a shrine to Sister Genevieve for bringing them the idea. As World War II unfolded, the male students quickly left, headed to far-flung sites to join the war effort. Enrollment plummeted to less than 100 students. During this time, a large percentage of graduates from the University of Portland were nurses whose numbers had soared because of the war. The priests could never have envisioned that it would be the nurses who kept the university financially afloat during this challenging time.

TRIAL ADMITTANCE

Dee had been brought up with as much privilege as possible, given she was the daughter of Italian immigrants who counted their pennies. Dee had beautiful clothes, even though she didn't care about that sort of thing. Her mother Theresa cared, though, remembering her teen days fondly when she and Dorothy would dress up in her best clothes. Theresa made sure her petite daughter—now a beautiful woman, with masses of black wavy hair, a big smile and an hourglass figure—was decked out in the latest fashion, even if there was a war going on. Theresa's own career at the bank thrived, and she thought office work would be perfect for her beautiful daughter when she graduated high school. "Nice and safe," Theresa thought. It would allow her daughter to be independent and it wouldn't tax her heart.

Dee listened patiently to her mother waxing on poetically about office work, but remained steadfast in her decision to be a nurse. It was with that determination that Dee convinced her parents in 1942 to drive her up the hill for an interview to be admitted to the School of Nursing.

Dee checked off the nursing school's requirements in its admissions brochure:

1. Graduate from an accredited high school: check
2. Stand academically in the top half of your class: check
3. Successful completion of the Nursing Aptitude Test: would be a cinch once she was admitted, she thought: check
4. Pleasing personality: well double check, thought Dee
5. Integrity of character: of course, check
6. Sympathetic understanding of people: check!

Frank, always the peacemaker, just wanted his daughter to be happy, and he convinced Theresa it was time to give in on this decision. Theresa was afraid of the physical toll nursing would take on her daughter, but she grudgingly agreed to the interview at least. She silently hoped that her daughter would either change her mind or, if not, meet some nice doctor during her training and carve a secure future for herself where she didn't have to work.

The three of them drove across town for an interview with Sister Genevieve. Despite being petite, Sister Genevieve was an imposing figure. She carried herself with dignity, decked out in a full black habit that overtook her entire head, while framing her face in a unique roll that was the visible trademark of the Sisters of Providence.

Known for her unselfish and untiring graciousness, she looked Dee over critically, however, clearly concerned. Sister Genevieve commented that the 5-foot-2, 110-pound girl didn't look like she could do the job very effectively.

Despite her reluctance for Dee to become a nurse, Theresa fixed her black eyes steadily on the nun. "She's young and stronger than she looks," Theresa said with conviction, her body language silently daring the nun to argue. And with that, Dee found herself admitted to the St. Vincent School of Nursing. Sister Genevieve left her with the caveat, though: "We will give her six months, and if she can't keep up, she will have to go." Theresa merely lifted her chin, stared the nun down, not flinching, silently accepting the challenge. Despite the warnings from the doctor and her own lack of enthusiasm for nursing, Theresa rose to the occasion, completely confident in her daughter's abilities and inner strength. More importantly, if this was truly her daughter's dream, then Theresa would move heaven and earth to ensure Dee was going to get the opportunity to achieve it.

As with any incoming student, however, Dee would have to be examined by a physician at the cost of $10, have a dental examination, chest X-ray and the required inoculations.

As a freshman and Portland resident, Dee could have been admitted as a day student, traveling back and forth up the hill each day. It may have been the wasted time it would take each day traveling on the streetcar or the desire not to have nightly conversations about her career choice with her mother, that helped Dee make the decision that she wanted to live in the Nurses' Home adjacent to the hospital.

As Dee prepared to leave home, she placed her suitcase on her painted iron twin bed, now a faded blue with little roses on the headboard. As she packed, Theresa appeared at the door. She held a bulky flour sack that had been bleached and recycled into a dishcloth. In it appeared to be a large object. Theresa sat down across from Dee on the other twin bed, which once had been Trixie's. Time had gotten away from her, and now her Dee was embarking on her own adventure. Theresa took off her thick trifocals, her black eyes a little misty. She quickly wiped her eyes with her usual handkerchief that she kept in her apron pocket, then placed her glasses back on her nose smartly. Theresa thrust the large object to Dee without a word. Unwrapping it, Dee found a bottle of whiskey. "For emergencies," said Theresa, in a tone that cautioned no refusal. Dee added it to her open suitcase with a smile.

"Thanks, Mom."

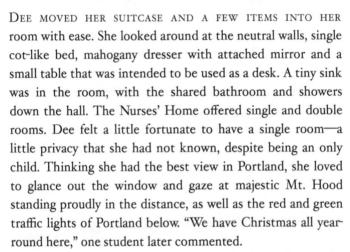

DEE MOVED HER SUITCASE AND A FEW ITEMS INTO HER room with ease. She looked around at the neutral walls, single cot-like bed, mahogany dresser with attached mirror and a small table that was intended to be used as a desk. A tiny sink was in the room, with the shared bathroom and showers down the hall. The Nurses' Home offered single and double rooms. Dee felt a little fortunate to have a single room—a little privacy that she had not known, despite being an only child. Thinking she had the best view in Portland, she loved to glance out the window and gaze at majestic Mt. Hood standing proudly in the distance, as well as the red and green traffic lights of Portland below. "We have Christmas all year-round here," one student later commented.

Dee didn't have time to settle in, as she skipped down the stairs for orientation with Miss Harriett Osborn. Dee knew the students were expected to pray, learn, and work under her guise. Dee sat perfectly still, a little in awe of Miss Osborn's presence, listening to her outline her expectations.

A tall woman who stood erect, Harriett had dark, short, wavy hair and a no-nonsense approach. Harriett would never have been described as beautiful, but there was something about her that held a person's attention. She had expressive, captivating eyes under dark eyebrows, and despite her stern approach, a beautiful smile with deep dimples. She was once portrayed as simply having "a unique humanness." Harriett wore a revised uniform of the student nurses, heavily starched, of course. Harriett's cap was always straight, her uniform spotless.

Ozzy (a nickname the student nurses would soon learn and only dare to whisper behind her back) walked the halls with grace and dignity, and a sharp eye that took in every detail with just one glance. "There's always a need for well-prepared nurses," Ozzy once wrote and she dedicated her life to ensuring there was no short supply—at least under her watch.

Life in the Nurses' Home was strict and methodical. The students' studies were rigorous and the work at the hospital was backbreaking, warned Ozzy. At the end of their hard work, four-year students would receive a diploma—something Ozzy was very proud of.

Ozzy told the students she would perform daily inspections: student nurses' hair was to be off the collar, no lipstick was allowed. Jewelry of any kind was forbidden.

The rules were made very clear: Students had to be in by 10:30 p.m. each night on the weekend and during the summer; 10 p.m. Monday, Tuesday, Wednesday and Thursday. Once a month, the students were allowed one overnight privilege or to have a later curfew of 12:30 a.m. (for freshmen, this was allowed only on weekends). Seniors were living the high life, receiving nine 1 a.m. curfews a month. The girls signed in with the exact time when arriving back from their late leave. A separate sheet of paper was even placed out for anyone coming in after 12:30 a.m. so they could be easily identified.

If a student's GPA dropped below 2.0, she was only allowed four privileges a month. Special extensions were given for certain occasions, such as basketball games, concerts, holidays and balls. If students were attending the

Senior Ball, they could roll in at 2 a.m. without a backward glance.

Any special leaves required a permit. This could be granted in the case of illness of a student, or serious illness or death of an immediate family member. However, students were not allowed to go home to take care of sick friends or relatives.

Checks or demerits were issued for breaking some of the rules. The girls were given "on campus status," which meant they must be in by 10 p.m. for one week if they had three checks/demerits in a week. The checks were given for:

1. An untidy room
2. Nonattendance at morning prayer, unless working nights or on a day off
3. Nonattendance at convocation, or assembly
4. Appearing on the elevator below the second floor in anything but street clothes or uniform
5. For every five minutes late, they received one check
6. For being 30 minutes late, students would receive a two-week sentence
7. For being 45 minutes late, students would receive a three-week sentence
8. For being an hour late, students would receive a month sentence

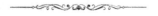

DEE FOLLOWED THE OTHER FRESHMEN OUT OF THE orientation, a little nervous and giddy at the same time. She glanced around and saw her classmates all had a timid look to them as they took in their surroundings.

The Nurses' Home was a bustling place, with student

nurses going in and out of its imposing front doors. While its lobby was nondescript, the T-Room was essentially a recreation room with ping-pong tables, piano, radio and even a record player.

On the first floor, the building featured an auditorium, library, reception room and a formal parlor for teas and dinners. Girls were forbidden from appearing on the first floor in jeans, slacks, bathrobes, housecoats or similar attire to ensure "gracious living," according to the admissions brochure.

A ramp led to the hospital's third floor. While nurses were encouraged to use it, they were urged to be quiet, so as not to disturb the patients.

A gym was available on the third floor of the Nurses' Home, where students could shoot baskets and even have a co-ed dance occasionally; all floors had a lounge for the students to congregate. Smoking was allowed in the T-room, reception rooms and the parlor where students could entertain a guest.

Way down in the basement, the laundry room with a wringer machine was found swishing clothes. Nursing students often held guard over the machine, enjoying a small corner to study before pairing up to drag their clothes through the wringer.

Dee soon learned Frances Rodgers was a mainstay at the switchboard which contained a complex buzzer system that was used to signal the students if they had a telephone call, a visitor, or were wanted on duty. One buzz was a phone call where the girls would race to the phone closet and pray no one was using it so they could accept their call. Two buzzes meant excitement—a visitor—students would often fly down the stairs two at a time to see who was there.

Frances Rodgers manned the sign-out book as if she was

General Patton himself. She also took messages for the student nurses, including the ones directing nurses to see Miss Osborn. The students soon found that nothing good usually came from those meetings. Ozzy was tough—though fair—and she expected nothing less than perfection from her nurses.

That night, the freshmen students went quietly to dinner at the cafeteria, known as the Beanery. The students would learn the Beanery would keep them well-fueled with mostly carbohydrates, and yes, beans.

Dee was now one of dozens of women who hoped to be part of the Class of 1946. She later would learn a high percentage of girls wouldn't graduate. Some were too challenged by organic chemistry, which was known to eliminate many students. Some women found out that nursing wasn't as glamourous as the brochures promised. Others mysteriously disappeared into the night, with Dee only learning later it was because they had been "discovered." Discovered meant that they were married—probably a quick wedding before their beau shipped out to war. Even with the caveat that no husband was actually present, marriage remained forbidden by the Sisters of Providence's student nurse requirements. Dee was sad to see some of her fellow student nurses leave simply because of a ridiculous requirement the nuns wouldn't bend on.

That evening Dee received her eight assigned uniforms, hitting at mid-calf, each practically standing up on their own with the starch that was used. Though the uniform was so stiff it crackled when she walked, Dee was very relieved the hospital had gone to a simplified version prior to her arrival. The long pinstriped uniforms with huge white aprons had now been hung up for this contemporary model that sported a Peter Pan collar, thick buttons, and the St. V's crest over the students' hearts. When they traveled outside the hospital, the nurses wore navy blue capes with bright red lining with gold STV embroidered on the collars.

The uniforms were worn with white silk hose—with garter belts (pantyhose had not been invented yet). However, the war effort was taking all the material used for women's stockings to make parachutes. The nursing students became adept in cultivating store clerks who would call them when the scarce hose came in, whispering into the phone and speaking cryptically, as if they were conducting an intricate spy deal as part of the war effort. An underclassman would soon be dispatched down to the drugstore to buy hose in every size for her classmates, who would then undertake the tedious task of dying them white.

Dee tried on the hose that featured seams in the back. Dee's seams would somehow end up always twisted around, zigzagging around her legs—leaving her tugging at them in a frustrated manner. On her feet she wore sturdy Army-type white shoes that had to be hand polished to keep their appearance. She would soon learn that Ozzy would even bend down from her impressive height, peering closely to ensure the shoelaces on those sturdy shoes were clean, and no dirt clung to them.

Dee was eager to make friends. She was also a bit nervous. Dee had heard rumors about secret initiations in the classes before her—where girls were blindfolded and forced to dip their hands in something scary or gross by the upperclassmen. There were stories about initiations where the seniors would share tales of the ghosts that wandered the halls. Freshmen before her were initiated by drinking out of what they later learned were unused urinals. Fortunately for Dee and her fellow freshmen, Ozzy was on to these shenanigans and there was no hazing such as this to be had.

Dee met Muriel first, who lived next door. Muriel's and Dee's mother had similar ideas about how to send off their daughters, only Muriel brought champagne. That champagne didn't last, as the girls gathered to drink it and kick off their freshman year. The girls would later congregate often in Dee's room, and others, to share secrets and laughter about everything they encountered during their shift. Dee soon learned her single room would be filled with girls, and suddenly that privacy she sought seemed to not be worth it. She was used to noise and lots of people; she found living, learning, praying and working in this bustling atmosphere to be ideal. The more noise the better, Dee thought, especially when it came to laughter and fun.

Dee quickly became close with two students: Annabelle, a tall, slender girl from nearby Beaverton, Oregon, who loved to laugh and get silly; and Sybil, a sweet, hardworking girl with masses of curly blond hair. The three pledged to stick together through classes, endless shifts, and rotations through each specialty.

The days and nights were also filled with unforgettable fun and laughter. Still, they had no idea what they were in for.

THE PATIENT COMES FIRST

D ee filed into her religion class, moving slowly after morning chapel at 6 a.m. She had barely kept her eyes open at chapel, trying to focus instead on the elaborate altar, with its tall candles and the statue of the Pietà that gleamed from above. To keep herself awake, she counted the beautiful stained-glass windows that lined the chapel as sunlight glinted through, creating an array of colors.

Dee had to smile when she remembered how she wasn't the only one who was sleepy. The non-Catholic girls were especially bleary-eyed, as they were not used to Catholic mass. They glanced around to see what everyone else was doing, robotically getting to their knees, their lips moving cautiously, though in reality nothing came out of their mouths. As they stood, the students' knees often caught on their calf-length starched uniforms. They stifled their giggles as Ozzy turned around, one eyebrow raised.

The days would have a rhythm. Chapel, inspection, breakfast, floor duty until 11, scurrying up the stairs to St. Theresa Hall for class until 3 p.m. and then back to floor duty until 7 or 8 p.m. The younger students were expected to work up to

42 practical hours while also studying. The nuns cautioned the 42 hours was a varying number, that there may be some cause for it to be irregular because of emergencies. If so, the school brochure reiterated this mandate and said the girls were to meet these expectations, "cheerfully and willingly." The nursing students dropped exhausted into their beds, whether it was at night or the morning, depending on what shift they worked.

Gone were the days where classes were taught by just the sisters and possibly a doctor they could scrounge up. Now, just a few of the sisters were involved in teaching. Instructors included physicians, as well as nursing school graduates who had been specially sought and recruited by Ozzy. With the university now actively involved, six priests and professors were also summoned up the hill to teach nonmedical subjects, such as English and of course, religion. All Catholic students were required to take religious studies during their freshman and sophomore years. Non-Catholic students were not required, but strongly *encouraged*.

Dee enjoyed her classes, absorbing the knowledge, especially science. As with most classes, the students sat alphabetically and the three R's—Rennie, Read and Richter—were perched in the back. The three weren't particularly good friends, but they were bonded by alphabetical seating and, of course, thankful they could hide from whoever was teaching, especially the priests, who were often dry as dust. One priest, Father Scanlan, took pity on some of the students, especially the older ones, whose fatigue was showing from working nights. Father Scanlan purposely didn't have a seating chart, but simply took one look at those who were working long hours and pointed to the back of the class. In the end, he felt better having his students fall asleep in the back of the room, rather than in the row right in his sightline.

Unknowingly, Dee sat in the front row one morning,

rubbing her eyes. The girls had kept her up late the night before gossiping and laughing. Father Scanlon's voice had a monotone quality and Dee rested her chin on her elbow, blinking her eyes rapidly. She glanced over at Annabelle who was using her fingers to literally prop her eyes open. Laughing to herself, Dee adjusted, squirming in her chair. Eventually, Father Scanlon's lecture got the best of her and Dee's eyes closed ever so briefly—or so she thought!

"Miss Rennie, do you have the answer? Miss Rennie?" droned the priest. Dee woke up with a start as Annabelle kicked her in the shin.

"I didn't hear the question, Father," said Dee politely. "I was asleep," she added honestly. The annoyance on the priest's face was evident as the class snickered.

A hand shot up across the room. "Miss Encyclopedia of the World," as Dee and Annabelle had already nicknamed her, was ready and willing to answer the question for Dee. As with life's irony, Betty was book smart, but not people smart. She took pride in correcting people—or as she referred to it as, "plain speaking." She was the one who would point out to a fellow student that she had a run in her stockings, or forgot to pin her hair up, provoking anger and rolling eyes from her classmates. Dee wondered what kind of nurse she'd make— maybe a better teacher, she thought. Betty reportedly got the best grades in the class, but was inept on the floor, incapable of even making a patient comfortable or showing much compassion. In the meantime, Betty answered Father Scanlon's question extensively, smirking across the room at Dee. Never one for much of a poker face, Dee pasted a fake smile on her face in return.

Dee's next class also featured a priest, but she never fell asleep in his class. Father John Hooyboer, who taught English, was popular among the students. The Reverends John and Cornelius "Con" Hooyboer were brothers who looked remarkably alike with their thin, balding hair and round wire-rim glasses perched on their large noses. The tall, lanky priests originally hailed from the Netherlands and had been educated at Notre Dame before moving on to the seminary. Father John, the older of the two, had first set out for Portland in the 1930s and became deeply devoted to the university. After his brother Con joined him, the two became known as "The Dutch Masters" on the Bluff.

Father John appreciated the university's affiliation with the nursing school on a personal level. He once discussed how his father had an appendicitis after the family moved from North Holland to the Midwest in the United States. It was 1917, and because of the lack of medical facilities, a doctor performed the operation on the patriarch of the family using the kitchen table. The wound never healed correctly and one day his father died after working in the fields on their family farm. From then on, Father John was a big fan of medical facilities and felt honored to be teaching future caregivers.

As was typical with him, Father John took on too many responsibilities. He shuttled back and forth to teach the student nurses English and religion, always late, running up the stairs of St. Theresa Hall, adjusting his spectacles and sailing into class. He had a legendary memory, calling each student by name. If Father John knew you, he knew you for life.

In fact, he appeared to know Dee even before she started attending his class. On the first day, she had walked in, eager to grab a seat next to Annabelle. She had heard Father John was a little disorganized and didn't enforce a seating chart. When Dee walked in, however, Father John pointed to a chair. "You sit here, Miss Rennie. I've heard about you." Dee watched in frustration as he pointed to the farthest seat away from Annabelle, who dutifully sat down in her designated seat, grinning and making a face at Dee behind Father John's back.

Today, Father John began handing out a simple assignment for the students to complete. Bending over her paper, Dee watched as Marcy settled into a chair by her. Though a nice girl, Marcy was constantly chewing—wads of paper, gum, virtually anything she could fit into her mouth. Dee watched in fascination as she walked in late as always, chewing away.

Ultimately, the instructor always demanded she spit it out, but as Dee tried to focus on her paper, she realized Father John must have a high tolerance for noise because he had not instructed Marcy to stop chewing.

As Dee filled out her paper, all she could do was count the number of chews. Chew, chew, chew. Silence. Chew. She's not even in rhythm, Dee sighed. Now completely unfocused, she glanced over and saw Miss Encyclopedia diligently filling out her paper easily. Dee bent back down to her paper and counted chews until she turned in what she was sure was not a very well-written assignment. Fortunately, it was just English, shrugged Dee. She cared more about her science and nursing classes.

The classes themselves were laborious, and included: anatomy and physiology, the dreaded organic chemistry, general psychology, history of nursing and even pathogenic bacteriology. This was in addition to English, PE and their religion classes. And that was just the first year.

Sophomores focused on nutrition, pharmacology, principles of medical and surgical nursing, neurology and urological nursing. Dermatology, communicable diseases, geriatrics and gynecology were also instructed. Dee longed for sophomore year when she would also learn operating techniques.

Junior year, the students would learn about orthopedics, obstetrics, ethics, pediatrics and psychology nursing.

Fourth year was centered on clinical experience with rotations in a variety of environments.

Guest lecturers were brought in as often as possible, and some classes were just a few hours. Part of the agreement with the University of Portland was the school would produce well-rounded nurses. To fulfill this, in addition to the medical instruction, the girls even attended classes on such subjects as political science, U.S. government, sociology and public speaking.

The students often studied in their rooms. Late at night, they sat at their wooden desks, groggy and often distracted by lights below. They made use of the expansive library in the Nurses' Home, studying as long as they could without being ultimately distracted by one of their friends. Frequently, someone would appear to coerce these studious women into a late-night feast or the idea to explore the hospital's basement just in case the ice cream bar—that would magically appear without warning—was operating.

The students focused on their studies, but knew they would be learning the most in those ever-present practical hours. Sister Genevieve and Ozzy had directed that nurses would evolve from disease-centered to patient-centered. "The patient comes first," Ozzy repeated over and over until the girls heard that phrase in their dreams.

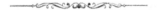

DEE COULDN'T WAIT TO GET OUT OF THE CLASSROOM AND have hands-on training. However, her idea of hands-on was more exciting than her first experience. For three months, the students endured training in how to sterilize equipment properly. Sister Georgette Bayless was nothing if not thorough. Dee rocked back on her heels, trying to eye the clock discretely, as Sister droned on, often repeating herself, knowing the students were taking in only some of the information.

Syringes were boiled and autoclaved. The students soon learned everything was autoclaved, including stainless steel bedpans, drinking water pitchers and emesis basins (used for patients who needed to vomit).

Worse was the bedpan flusher, thought Dee, grimacing. Though it was meant to make life easier, often a student struggled with the contraption. Frequently, its lid would not close and the attached water hose was bulky and prone to leaking.

The very next day, the students learned the challenges of that particular flusher, involving a certain girl by the name of Ann Smith. Ann was a Portland girl, and was tall, slim and had dark hair and distinct straight bangs. She loved to laugh and was very popular among all the students.

As Dee walked by during her shift that next morning, she saw Ann in the Hopper Room with the bedpan flusher. Ann flashed her wide smile and bent to her task. She was struggling to close the lid and as usual, the temperamental device took over. Dee suddenly heard a loud scream and came running back to see Ann covered in human waste. Dee's eyes widened, not sure what to do as Ann looked at her in horror. And then Ann did something simply remarkable: She began to laugh. Clutching her stomach, Ann laughed until she cried. Dee hung on to the doorframe, laughing as well. Their laughter rang out through the halls and without warning, Ozzy appeared. She walked over and peered into the doorway, raised one eyebrow, sighed, and simply walked away.

Meanwhile, Ann and Dee discussed how this incident sparked newfound knowledge about the flusher and how it might create an opportunity for them in the future. That plan would develop over the coming months. Soon, rigging the bedpan flusher to spray some unfortunate younger student nurse became an art form and one generally employed by Dee's classmates. It was all in great fun, they rationalized, just as long as Ozzy didn't catch you.

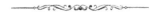

THE STUDENTS SOON LEARNED THE AUTOCLAVE AND sterilization were trying, but giving a hypo (shot) was even more so. Dee skipped into class that day, excited about learning how to administer a syringe. She couldn't wait to try giving a shot.

After Sister Bayless' lengthy explanation, Dee wasn't so sure she wanted to know anymore. No one would ever describe Dee as methodical, which meant she had to summon up every bit of patience to please the exacting nun during class. The nursing students were instructed to boil the hypo needle and syringe in a small container over a Bunsen burner for three minutes, and then lay the needle end on an alcohol-soaked chunk of cotton. They then boiled water in a spoon, popped the drug—whether it was morphine, codeine or other drugs—into the syringe, drew up the boiling water to 1 cc and shook the hypo to dissolve its contents. From there, they could gloriously march off to relieve a suffering patient—in this case, they sort of pretended it was each other—stopping short, of course, of giving the actual shot.

Three months were also spent learning how to scrub instruments. The student nurses were taught to use ether to sterilize everything. Students who didn't follow directions fainted on the floor with the smell of the highly flammable ether they were using to sterilize. Sister just shook her head, instructing a couple of students to make the prone girl on the floor comfortable and let her come to on her own.

Next, Sister taught them how to sharpen the needles. With wide eyes, Dee looked around and watched the others.

As always, Annabelle wiggled her eyebrows at her and Dee dissolved into giggles, dropping her needle. Sister walked over to ask if she was done and Dee scrambled to grab her now-contaminated needle, obediently telling the nun that no, she wasn't quite finished yet.

And they weren't done. The next lesson was how to make a solution for an IV, while also making sure they sterilized the tubing that would be recycled and reused. Dee wondered at this point if she was going to actually help people or make them sicker!

The students soon learned the most wearisome part of the entire process was actually trying to find a match for the Bunsen burners. Matches were scarce during wartime. The sisters kept these rare matches under lock and key, and it added a layer of frustration to locate one (and God forbid if two were actually needed) to complete the task.

Rounding out their instruction were eminent physicians by the names of Sommer, Joyce, Sabin, Meienberg and Gilmore. They were responsible for some of the instruction, especially the hands-on teaching of the young student nurses. This group of older gentlemen, elegantly garbed in their dapper suits and bowler hats, demanded respect and were known to berate a nursing student for not getting to all of her 20 patients in a timely manner. Once in a while, the doctors would be accompanied by young residents who would breeze through the wards, learning rapidly from the experienced doctors before going off to war. These young men ran behind them, carrying the doctors' papers and bags, and tending to their needs. The nurses and nursing students were required to stand in a doctor's presence, even if he walked in unannounced to the chart room. The nursing students were taught to answer their rapid questions succinctly and write any additional orders down accordingly. The nurses and students were commanded to address them by "sir" or "doctor."

Dee watched as Dr. Joyce, head of surgery, performed his daily round. Accompanied by a large entourage, he toured the ward, barking orders at her and the other students. Exhausted, Dee continued to care for her patients, taking care that Ozzy didn't see her roll her eyes at the usual arrogance of the doctor's expectations.

The next morning, Dee arrived on the floor for her first assignment and followed her orders to check in with the sister in charge. She quickly found Sister Clementia to tell her she had arrived from chapel. As was routine, the students were assigned four patients to bathe and then change their bed linens. The students cranked up the beds and heaved heavy patients by themselves around the bed so they could perform these tasks. They would then sweep the floor and rugs, dust, and refresh flowers of anyone who was fortunate to have received them. After that was done, it was time to take TPRs—temperature, pulse and respirations—give medications and carry out any additional orders from the doctors, answer call lights, and empty bedpans and urinals. And that was all before 10 a.m., when charting was also to be finished.

Then it was on to class only to come back and focus on delivering any leftover lunches that hadn't been given, or carrying the trays back out if they hadn't been cleared. On top of meals, the nursing students were responsible for morning and midafternoon nourishment of juices. Glasses and water pitchers were collected, washed, dried, refilled with ice water and returned to each bedside table. Not more liquid, thought Dee, for she knew patient intake and output would have to be measured and charted. And of course, that meant more bedpans!

In the morning and afternoon, there was wheelchair time for patients who were allowed up, most taking two nurses to get a patient into a chair. It seemed like mere minutes passed before it was time to heave them back into bed.

There was always something happening—going over instructions before leaving her shift, making new admissions comfortable, listening to a patient's loved ones—quietly comforting them as if she had all the time in the world. It was never-ending and Dee loved it.

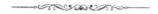

IT WAS A QUIET DAY ON THE WARD. THE PATIENTS WERE roaming in their wheelchairs, some casually conversing with others.

As Dee finished her charting, she heard the familiar click-click down the hall and knew in just a matter of moments Dr. Boyden would reach her.

"Good afternoon, Miss Rennie," he barked.

"Dr. Boyden," she acknowledged, trying not to laugh. Dr. Boyden had just recently arrived at St. Vincent after serving in Sicily and Normandy. He had been awarded a Bronze Star, but was humble and encouraging to the students.

Despite being one of the students' favorites, they had to giggle when they heard him "click, click, click" down the hall.

I hope he didn't wear those shoes in the war, thought Dee. The enemy would have heard him coming for sure.

Dee went to tell Sybil her new joke, since they both had time on their hands. Looking around, Dee sensed what was going to occur. When the days slowed such as this, the nuns looked around and found busywork for the students. In this case, it usually meant ordering them off to the Hopper Room to sterilize bedpans. When Dee found Sybil, it was obvious her friend was trying to appear busy in an attempt to ward off what they both knew was coming.

"Sister, why don't I go pick up the afternoon prescriptions?" asked Sybil innocently, trying not to look at Dee's indignant face.

Sister glanced up from her charting and nodded. She turned to Dee and her kind eyes saw the dread.

"You can go with her, Miss Rennie," she said, eyes twinkling. "When you get back, you both can make quick work of the bedpans."

The girls took off laughing, for it was always a race to the Central Pharmacy. The student nurses knew the stairs were faster than the elevator. The stairs, gleaming from constant polishing by the janitorial staff, were slippery and the girls could almost slide down the stairs in one steady motion in their thick white shoes.

On this day, Sybil was faster, outpacing Dee readily. Dee caught up as they neared the pharmacy and now they were running, with Sybil in the lead. They rounded the corner and slid the final few feet. Out of breath, Sybil, clearly the winner, jumped in victory. Dee bent over, laughing and out of breath. Sister Stanislaus, who oversaw the pharmacy, just watched the two, shaking her head, her sweet face surrounded by its white wimple.

Unfortunately, the way up wasn't quite as much fun, especially knowing the Hopper Room was waiting for them.

RESPECT THE CAP

Freshmen girls were lacking something at the St. Vincent School of Nursing. They enviously looked at the sophomores, juniors and seniors with a bit of wistfulness and longing. What was missing? The cap.

St. Vincent School of Nursing students didn't receive their caps until the first term of their sophomore year. Caps meant everything to the student nurses—it meant they were truly on their way to becoming a nurse. Its reverence was ingrained in the girls, so much so that once the students had one, it was used as a punishment of sorts. Get in trouble, make a mistake in front of a doctor or raise Ozzy's ire, and a student would be told to turn their cap in to Ozzy for a specified amount of time.

The cap was more than just a nurse's hat; it was a true sign of the women's dedication to the profession of nursing. The students learned early on that caps were a sacred part of the uniform. Adapted from early Christians and modified over the years after the Victorian era, caps had become a requirement for nurses around the world. St. Vincent nurses originally had round caps with frills and a black ribbon tied around it. That cap had evolved as well and now was a more traditional nurse's cap with a broad bottom and two points at the top. It was worn proudly at the crown of the nursing students' heads. Any graduate could be identified by her hat, a clear designation if she was local or not.

The Capping Ceremony was one of grand tradition that was so profound, the local newspaper wrote about the ceremony, naming each student to be honored. Students were provided invitations to send to loved ones. Parents came early to the St. Vincent Hospital Chapel to get good seats. The Sisters of Providence sat in the balcony, their white and black habits peeping over the ledge, keeping a watchful eye over their students.

As the students filed in solemnly to the hymn of "O God of Loveliness," the priests from the University of Portland waited on the altar. The students had the cap, essentially a white piece of starched white fabric lying flat on their heads, the ends trailing down behind them, almost like a small bridal veil. The students to be capped each had a "big sister," a senior who marched proudly in with them, taking their place next to their charge. Big sisters had the honor of folding the cap up and pinning it in place on their little sister's head at the appointed time during the ceremony. They would later have to learn how to fold and pin their caps after they were washed—a tedious procedure at first, but one soon they could do practically in their sleep.

Dee sat nervously, awaiting this complex procedure. She glanced over her shoulder, saw her parents and gave a small wave before dropping her hand as Ozzy gave her a stern look. The priest's sermon seemed to stretch on and on, until finally they stood to sing "Ave Maria," one of Dee's favorite hymns.

Dee's big sister, Terry Valentine, was an excellent match. Terry was even more petite than Dee and just as fiery. Terry didn't shy away from telling Dee what she needed to know.

Dee scrunched down slightly as Terry folded the cap upward, sticking white pins into Dee's black head of curls.

Upon completion of all the students' caps getting pinned up, they recited the "Fidelity to Duty" pledge and then sat down once again while Ozzy addressed the class and audience.

Dee said later she remembered little about the ceremony after she officially received her cap. She was too busy moving her head slowly around, wondering how many pins she would need to ensure it stayed firmly on her full head of hair. She marveled that it seemed light, but at the same time, almost added a weight of responsibility.

One thing Dee remembered, however, was the last thing Ozzy said at the podium before taking her seat again.

"Nurses, always remember this: Respect the cap."

MISCHIEF MAKING

Rosemary liked men. A classmate of Dee's, she was a beautiful girl who became known early on for her love of a good time. Since it was wartime, most men—well, men who women would actually *want* to date—were gone, long shipped off to fight in the war. That didn't stop Rosemary. She brushed her glossy black hair, donned her finest dress, dug out some nice hose with seams and strapped on a pair of spiky black heels. Remarkably, even with those four-inch heels on, she could still snake down the fire escape at the back of the building, disappearing quickly into the night to go meet a new beau. Dee shook her head, watching Rosemary's demerits stack up, as she was usually caught sneaking back in late at night. Three demerits and a student's overnight privileges were snapped up by Ozzy. "I'd rather lose my cap," thought Dee, then to explain to her mother why she wasn't allowed to come home.

However, on this particular night, Dee and some of the girls followed Rosemary's lead down the fire escape—not to meet men—but to travel covertly down to nearby Northwest 23rd Avenue. Their destination was Henry Thiele's, a famed

Portland restaurant that stood proudly at an awkward intersection where several streets met jaggedly at the corner of Northwest 23rd and Westover. Its back room was often filled with St. V's student nurses, who gathered to smoke, drink and chat the night away.

Later that night, the women were hurrying home after a fun time, laughing with each other. They were running on Westover toward the hospital when a man staggered by, drunkenly exposing himself to the surprised group. Their eyes wide, they stopped dead in their path.

"I've seen better," shouted Annabelle. The girls shrieked with a combination of horror and laughter. They tried to contain themselves quickly, but the commotion made them even later than they had hoped. The women ran again, trying to get home desperately before bed check. Bed check began promptly at 10 p.m. each night for the student nurses and Tillie Erickson, the housemother, went methodically from room to room, opening and closing the students' doors as quietly as she could, shining her metal flashlight to guide her as she went.

As the girls climbed the fire escape upon their return, their giggles drowned out only by their constant shushing each other, they knew they were cutting it close. Tillie might be on their floor by now. It was possible, they thought, to just sail into the corner room directly from the fire escape unnoticed. From there, they could convince her they were just mingling in a friend's room and had lost track of time. Never mind that they all smelled of liquor and cigarettes, they thought the plan still had merit.

"Hello, Sister!" the group suddenly heard Dee say cheerfully, as if she was trying to portray them climbing up the fire escape late at night as a normal occurrence. The other five girls' heads snapped up immediately, their eyes trapped in the light. Sister Genevieve, flashlight in hand, stood at the window Dee was about to climb into. Sister stepped aside quietly, her face stern in its oval habit. As the girls silently followed Dee in, they glanced quickly at Sister Genevieve before scurrying to their rooms. Not a word was said until the next day after chapel when, as expected, notes addressed to the fire escapees were all lined up in tidy order at the base of Frances Rodgers' switchboard. Each said the same thing:

"Please leave your cap at the desk." Harriett Osborn, RN, BSN

Dee grimaced, unpinning her cap, and resignedly handed it to Frances Rodgers.

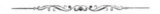

THE FIRE ESCAPE OFFERED OPPORTUNITY FOR OTHERS AS well, but not in a good way. One night, Dee, Annabelle, Sybil and a few others were sitting in a students' rooms near the fire escape. Yawning and talking quietly, they mended their hose, polished their shoes and gossiped about their day.

"What was that?" shrieked two of the women suddenly, standing up, pointing outside.

"What?" the others asked calmly with a yawn, used to the dramatics routinely surrounding them.

"A man! A man is on the fire escape!" the students shouted, convinced they had seen the outline of a male figure peering into a window.

The group sprung to their feet, tying their bathrobes, and hastily began grabbing baseball bats, tennis rackets, shoes, and anything they could find. Students emerged from their rooms to see what the fuss was about. Screaming commenced, and the small group became a larger one in seconds.

With bathrobes on, curlers in their hair and slippers on their feet, the women jumped out the window on to the fire escape, chasing the man downward. He glanced upward at the advancing throng of angry screeching women, and stepped up his retreat, taking the stairs two and three at a time. At the bottom, he ran off into the shadows of the night, eastward down the sloping hill, away from the hospital, glancing back frantically to make sure he wasn't being followed. The throng continued, powered by pure adrenalin, disappointed they didn't get to use their homemade weapons on the intruder. The students abruptly stopped at the hospital driveway and slowly began walking back up the slope, indignant at the man's gall, chattering and laughing nervously.

As they got to the steps of the Nurses' Home, they saw Sister Genevieve, her black habit blending into the shadows, her arms crossed, her mouth quivering.

"Well, it's a good thing you didn't catch him or he would have been one of our patients," she said with a twinkle in her eye. And with that, she turned and filed in, with the still-frustrated crowd following slowly behind her, for once breaking the rule of no pajamas on the first floor. They didn't think Sister would mind just this once.

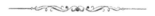

MAYBE IT WAS BECAUSE THEY WORKED SO HARD, BUT IF there was mischief to be made, the student nurses found a way to make it.

One night, Dee was studying, sitting at her desk, glancing occasionally out her window. Suddenly, her nose twitched! Smoke?!

She ran into the hallway, which was already getting smoky. "Fire!" she yelled. Doors began opening and alarmed girls ran into the hallway. Some were in bathrobes, while others were still in their uniforms, having just gotten off duty. The smoke was starting to curl into the hallway. Wildly, the girls took to the stairs and the fire escape, clamoring to get out of the home, shrieking as they went.

The girls lined up outside, shivering, as the fire trucks slowly made their way up the hill, sirens shattering the silence of the evening.

The sisters ran from student to student, checking in with each one, eager to ensure everyone was fine. Sister Genevieve had a clipboard, checking off the students, trying to determine who should be there and who was on duty.

"Where's Inarose?" asked Sister Genevieve to the crowd in general.

"I'm not sure, Sister," said one student. "Maybe she's still on duty."

"Oops," said another student, covering her mouth with a hand, her eyes darting between a look of alarm and a bit of humor.

In fact, Inarose *was* still inside. She was taking a nice, long shower on the fifth floor. It had been a tough day, and she had longed for this moment. Getting ready to step out, she grabbed for her towel, her hand hitting the bar at different places, and finding nothing. She wiped the water from her eyes and glanced around for it, thinking it had fallen to the floor, but there was nothing.

Wiping her bright red hair away from her face, she glanced over at the dresser where she had left her robe. Nothing.

It was not long before she heard the firemen's voices advancing on the floor.

No one knows what Inarose said that day, but they imagined that it might not have been something to repeat in front of the sisters. And they knew most certainly, it contained an element of revenge.

As for the smoke, no one quite remembered what started the small fire that did little damage. They remembered quite vividly, however, the fire in Inarose's eyes when they filed back in.

———❦———

DEE WAS EXHAUSTED. COMING OFF A 12-HOUR WORK SHIFT, she couldn't hold her eyes open any longer. Clad in a long warm nightgown, she got into bed, drew the covers up and was instantly asleep.

Dee was having the loveliest dream. She was floating slowly. She felt herself moving even slower, drifting downward. She turned over, sighed deeply, punching her pillow a little. She heard a slight ding and wondered if someone had a bell down the hall. Suddenly, she heard laughter. Who was in her dream? Who was laughing?

Annabelle had better not be coming to wake me up, she thought. If she does, I'm truly going to rig the bedpan flusher to blow up right in her face. Dee smiled at that thought.

The laughing continued. Opening her eyes reluctantly, she saw faces she knew.

Why are they in my dream? Dee thought, closing her eyes. The laughter got louder.

Opening her brown eyes even wider, she looked at the fingers pointing at her, and the faces—mouths open wide, emitting hysterical laughter.

Two doors drew together, blocking Dee's view. The ding came back and then she saw the girls again, now doubled over. Sitting up in bed, Dee looked around and then she realized where she was. Somehow, somewhere in the middle of the night, her friends had rolled her small bed into the elevator, folding the mattress ever so slightly and sending her on a vertical journey.

Flinging herself back into bed, Dee turned over. She'd deal with them later!

The next day, Dee found the expected note from Ozzy. It took all the control she had not to slam her cap down toward Frances Rodgers, feeling quite indignant at the unfair punishment for merely sleeping. Revenge would be sweet, she thought. She just had to think of something.

———◆———

IT WASN'T LONG BEFORE DEE WAS ABLE TO EXACT A revenge of some sort, but this form of retribution involved the upperclassmen. Seniors were nothing but a pain, thought Dee. They cut in line at the Beanery and demanded that the freshmen wake them up in the mornings. Never mind that when it was Dee's turn, she accidentally woke up the wrong seniors and got yelled at for her trouble.

The worst demand by seniors was their insistence on receiving supreme elevator privileges. It didn't seem to matter to them that younger students were running to get to work or class on time, or getting off work dead tired. The seniors proclaimed they had priority over the hospital elevators; if anyone younger was on them, the seniors could easily kick them off, no questions asked.

Mr. Klein and Mr. Meyers ran the two manual elevators at the hospital. They did their jobs well, operating the elevator controls, pulling back the gate and running the hospital staff and visitors up and down throughout the day. Their faces never portrayed the extensive knowledge they gained through listening to constant gossip, especially from the student nurses. They handled their jobs with the utmost of decorum, bidding the students good day and good night in their monotone voices.

On this particular day, Dee just wanted to get to class on time for once. Dee, Annabelle and Sybil got in the elevator, and Mr. Klein greeted them in his usual solemn manner. Since he didn't have a full car, he told the students he would be back soon, shuffling off slowly to get a drink from the nearby water fountain.

Dee looked into the hallway, watching him absentmindedly. Suddenly, she saw a large group of seniors coming and her eyes widened. The seniors, plus Dee and her friends, would not all be able to fit in the elevator. As they approached, it became apparent to Dee that she and her friends were about to be unceremoniously tossed out as usual.

Without a word, Dee lurched for the elevator door and its subsequent gate, closing it with a big clang. She grabbed the control wheel and directed the elevator downward. "Dee, what are you doing?" the girls cried in alarm.

"It's okay," Dee smiled widely, and tried to reassure them, but with all of them screaming at once, they didn't hear her.

Dee smoothly glided the elevator to the lobby floor, dragging the gate and door open noisily and letting her friends disembark, now with shaky legs. The girls laughingly crossed the way to St. Theresa Hall, running up the stairs to go to class, ready to tell their friends what Dee had done now. Word spread like wildfire by the next morning that Dee Rennie had circumvented the seniors' rights, and taken a joy ride in the elevator. Dee didn't bother sharing the knowledge that she knew how to operate an elevator after working for the summer at the University of Oregon Medical School. In fact, she considered herself a professional, she thought smugly.

Ozzy didn't agree, but the next day, Dee smiled as she willingly handed her cap to a perplexed Frances Rodgers.

THE ONLY WAY TO LEARN

"The only way to learn is to get in there and do it," proclaimed Ozzy. Knowing she was right, Dee and her fellow students, now upperclassmen, found themselves excited about rotating through all the departments. Eventually, they would rotate through obstetrics, pediatrics, surgery, dietary, public health, etc., all at St. Vincent Hospital. There were two courses that were not at the hospital: psychiatric training was held at the Oregon State Hospital in Salem, and pediatric training was held at the new Providence Hospital. The Sisters of Providence had been busy again, building a new hospital in 1941 to serve the east side of Portland across the Willamette River.

Rotations were usually about six weeks in each department. The students were expected to work two-week shifts on days (7 a.m. to 3 p.m.), swing (3 p.m. to 11 p.m.) and nights (11 p.m. to 7 a.m.). Exceptions were surgery, which was just day shift, and maternity, which had a split night shift that was dreaded for students who couldn't sleep on command.

MEDICAL

Dee and her fellow classmates were assigned first to the more mundane medical units. Medical was a boring starting point, thought Dee, who greatly anticipated surgery, already knowing in her heart she would love it. In the medical ward, Dee's patients mostly were afflicted with diabetes or respiratory issues, such as pneumonia. The medical floors were also full of men from the shipyards or lumberyards who had dermatitis, an allergic reaction to handling wood.

Many of the patients had chronic illnesses or were just plain elderly. Dee decided she didn't much care for medical. Too much death, she thought to herself, as she walked by a room and watched one nun pull a sheet over the third patient to die that day.

"Dee, come here," Sister Fausta said, knowing Dee was there without even turning around—a unique skill all the nuns seem to possess. Making the sign of the cross and finishing her prayer, Sister firmly told Dee, "You and Shirley need to take this man to the morgue. He has expired," she added needlessly. "But, Sister," Dee started and then abruptly closed her mouth. She knew everyone was busy, and Sister was eager to get the patient to a place where others did not have to view what might be the possible end to their own stay at the hospital.

Having already been summoned by Sister, Dee's classmate, Shirley, sailed in and the two students wheeled the man down the hall, fighting the stretcher the whole way. Many of the hospital's stretchers were in terrible shape with rusty, squeaky wheels that wouldn't move as they were supposed to, instead fighting to go in different directions. The two students went out the door and down the ramp toward the back of the hospital where the morgue was. Thinking it was creepy behind the hospital, Dee gave the stretcher an extra shove in an attempt to get the errand done quickly. At the same time, Shirley hit a bump, and the deceased patient flew from the stretcher on to the pavement, the sheet askew. Dee and Shirley stared at each other, their mouths open, their eyes wide.

"What do we do now?" asked Shirley.

"Well, pick him up!" said Dee in a no-nonsense way. Looking both ways, the two students grabbed and heaved, and eventually got the body back to the stretcher and to the morgue with no more mishaps.

They didn't glance up to the window or they would have seen Sister Genevieve watching. She made the sign of the cross, shook her head, and went back to her desk.

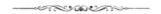

IT GOT EVEN WORSE THE NEXT DAY. OF ALL THE HOSPITAL wings, 2 North was the most notorious. It was the destination of many indigent men, who either lived in seedy hotels off nearby West Burnside Street or had been sent up by the city's jail. Some just needed detoxing, while others had been injured in a fight.

The night before, Dee heard that the nurses had a horrendous experience. A man was admitted who was at least 6-foot-4. He was found standing in the center of his bed trying to unscrew the ceiling light, an act which caused his hospital gown to become twisted, revealing everything the nursing students didn't want to see. All the men in the ward were laughing and pointing, "What are you girls going to do about this one?" The frightened student nurses stood there, riveted, their eyes huge. Finally, they just turned and ran.

The next day, things had gotten no better. Three students were attempting to wrestle with a different man, to no avail. Dee heard their shouts and headed in to help her friends.

Between the four of them, they wrestled the man down, stripped him, and scrubbed him clean. It was a job no one wanted, but the students all worked as fast as they could while holding their breaths at the same time.

"I want to go back to jail!" yelled the man.

"Whatever for?" asked Dee.

"They treat me better there," he grumbled.

Dee and the other students just looked at each other and shrugged. The student nurses started to clean up the resulting mess, one grabbing his clothes to put down the incinerator. The sisters kept a closetful of clean clothes from a variety of sources. When the patient was discharged, the sisters would outfit him in some castoff, clean clothes, as they usually did.

As the students prepared to leave the room, the patient suddenly panicked. He started to shake and climb out of his bed.

"You need to stay in bed," yelled Dee sharply.

The man continued to try desperately to stand on his shaky legs.

"You don't understand," he gasped. "I need my money! You took my clothes away to burn them and my money was in my..."

"Oh, you mean this?" Dee interrupted, grinning and holding up a dirty long sock with two fingers. "Don't worry. I've learned one thing already and that's where you guys keep your money." With that, she lobbed the sock onto his bed, her nose wrinkling.

The man laid back, content, counting his money, and Dee shook her head and washed her hands before tending to the next patient. She always remembered to look in the socks, no matter what.

DIETARY THERAPY

Sister Cresence ran the hospital's kitchen like an experienced general. Despite the organization, Dee thought dietary therapy was even more boring than the medical unit rotation. Sister had other ideas, droning on about the need for the low-sugar, low-fat diets for patients with diabetes, the soft diet for patients recovering from surgery, and more.

Dee stirred the hot cereal and yawned. If nothing else, this rotation was making her even more tired as well as hungry. She watched as her classmate, Dorothy Ann, lined up the crates that had just held oranges. With the oranges stored on the shelves, the crates were now stacked in the hallway, waiting for the janitor to find his way down to the kitchen to remove them. Dorothy Ann, who frequently reminisced about her days taking ballet lessons and her longing to be a ballerina, lined up the crates methodically, positioning them just so.

Dee's eyes widened in fascination as Dorothy Ann walked determinedly to the end of her line of crates, then backed up, a look of concentration on her face. Taking a running start, Dorothy Ann sailed over the first crate, her right leg ahead of her, her left straight behind her. She did the same for the next and the next, her long legs stretching in front and behind her in near perfect ballet form. Dorothy Ann cleared the last of them, a look of triumph on her face. Dee looked down at her short legs, shook her head and sighed.

"All this exercise is making me hungry," she told Dorothy Ann. Dee was already desperately tired of the Beanery. She was used to tantalizing Italian fare with fresh fruits and vegetables always on the table, and was gaining weight for the first time in her life. She glanced down at the buttons now pulling on the front of her uniform and prayed silently Ozzy wouldn't notice. Most of the older students had reported to

Dee they all gained weight initially, but endless hours as a floor nurse would soon take care of it.

Dee shrugged and figured she wasn't going to worry about the weight gain right now. She went to the freezer and took two dishes of ice cream off a tray that had been prepped for patients' lunches. Dorothy Ann laughingly came to join her. Glancing up, Dee saw that the ceiling tiles reflected down the hall.

"Quick—eat this and we'll watch for Sister in the ceiling tiles," Dee told Dorothy Ann, grabbing the dish of ice cream. As they gulped it down, they laughed, talking about how it hit the spot, even if it was 10 in the morning. Unfortunately, neither of them noticed Ozzy coming down the hallway from the other direction.

The note the next day by Frances Rodgers' switchboard was direct and to the point, as always: "Miss Rennie, please leave your cap at the switchboard. Harriett Osborn, RN, BSN"

SURGERY

Surgeries during the 1940s involved repairing appendices, gallbladders, fractures, thyroids, hernias or more involved colostomies, ileostomies and craniotomies. Recovery was difficult; patients who received appendectomies were hospitalized for at least 14 days and patients recovering from hernia surgeries were often hospitalized for three weeks.

Dee went into her first surgery with wide-eyed fascination. If Sister Cresence ran dietary like a general, then Sister Agnes must be a four-star general, thought Dee. Sister Agnes was sharp, to the point, and intolerant of any unprofessionalism in her operating rooms. Seeing that she had been there for so long, Dee knew it truly was considered her domain. She soon learned, though, that Sister Agnes was also patient and kind, often sending students and nurses off for free time, especially during the holidays while she covered for them. The doctors discovered they could make Sister Agnes giggle; two doctors in particular, Dr. Harry Blair and Dr. Herb Thatcher, were orthopedic men. They loved to tease Sister Agnes, playing little practical jokes when they could.

Surgery was an exhilarating place, with doctors sometimes racing—as safely as medically possible—on who could fix a hernia or an appendix faster, with Sister Agnes tut-tutting as they went.

Sister Agnes was also a teacher, always seeking quality equipment for training purposes, and finally acquiring surgical mannequins on which her students could practice. Patiently, she taught the students how to do a urinary catheterization. While Dee was not thrilled about performing this task, she framed it in her head as a surgical procedure, which allowed her to focus on the technique used. Sister patiently taught them to scrub their hands for five minutes and hold them aloft, while another nurse carried in the prepared tray, and draped the patient. Dee wrinkled her nose at the next part. A little shy in nature, threading a tube into a patient's urethra seemed at first to be an intrusion at the very least. Dee shrugged her shoulders and performed her first one nervously, but thankfully, successfully.

Later that day, Dee watched as Dr. E. St. Pierre, medical president of St. Vincent, walked erectly down the hall. An eminent surgeon, he was a tall, quiet, dignified man who had an unexpected fun side. Known simply as "The Saint," Dr. St. Pierre was revered.

On his way to the operating room to perform yet another surgery, he glanced around the seemingly empty hallway. Seeing no one about, he did a quiet little soft shoe dance, celebrating his most recent surgery: a tricky appendectomy. What he didn't realize was the nursing students often saw his soft shoe and looked forward to peeking around the corner and watching his post-surgery celebration.

Since Dee had completed the preparations for the surgery the night before, Sister Agnes allowed her to watch Dr. St. Pierre's next appendectomy. The tall man bent way over the patient, performing the surgery with practiced ease. As Dee watched the well-choreographed group in the operating room, she decided her calling was to become a surgical nurse.

This operation in particular became trickier than the Operating Room staff imagined, and the surgery took longer than usual. Dee, not used to standing still for that long, moved her weight to one foot and then the other, glancing at the old-fashioned clock as the hours ticked by. At last, Dr. St. Pierre was satisfied and the entire staff let out a collective sigh. Sister Agnes congratulated him on a successful surgery, despite the medical surprises he had dealt with.

Taking off his gloves and mask, he walked past Dee with a glimmer in his eye. "That's why they call me 'the Saint,'" he said with a smile to the surprised Dee, who tried desperately to keep from grinning behind her mask.

Dee waited for directions from Sister Agnes and followed the patient out of the Operating Room back to the ward. Recovery rooms were not yet a reality, so the student nurses were required to sit with each new surgical patient in the ward until he or she awoke from the anesthesia. Dee perched on her hard chair, alert at first, watching for any signs of distress. However, as usual, the residual sweet smell of the ether used as the anesthesia was so strong, she found her eyes drifting closed. Shaking herself, she walked around the room, trying to stay awake.

Dee thought back to the surgery and the excitement of it all. Placing her hands up to prop her eyelids opened, she smiled to herself. Surgery was the place to be.

PEDIATRICS

The "Principles of Pediatric Nursing" was a rotation Dee looked forward to since she loved children. She didn't like having to go across town to Providence Hospital, though, since that meant riding the street car all the way back to the Nurses' Home after an entire shift.

Pediatrics was certainly noisy and lively during the daytime, thought Dee, when she entered the ward later that week. The cheery wallpaper and the bright colors made for a festive atmosphere. Dee soon learned, however, that there was nothing worse than sick children. It bothered her to see these tiny humans flushed with fever, confused about where they were, and crying for their parents. The most common reason a child was hospitalized was for a tonsillectomy, which was a brutal surgery at the time and left the children in grave pain for days. Even the promised ice cream didn't bring a smile. Dee had heard stories of diphtheria also being found. One entire shift of nurses had to be tested and some quarantined following exposure.

Penicillin, a godsend, was being mass produced and distributed to hospitals. Dee was thrilled, knowing that if it had been invented and available when she was a young child, she would have avoided many of her grave illnesses. However, the penicillin was only available in three-hour doses and of course, had to be injected. That meant that the nurses would move through the ward injecting the penicillin; by the time they got to the other side, all the children were crying.

On this particular day, all was quiet. As Dee walked quickly down the hall, intent on visiting some of her favorite older children in the playroom, she glanced outside to see the rain. The sky was black, and the rain was driving down in sheets, hitting the hospital's windows with tiny pinging sounds. Suddenly, a crack of thunder was heard and the hospital's lights flickered. Dee cast an eye upward, frowning to herself. Sure enough, she heard a quick sizzle and then a zap, and the lights went out.

Sister suddenly rounded the corner, her skirt flapping behind her. If it wasn't for the worried look on her face, Dee would have laughed at her attempt to run in her full habit, the nun's wimple catching wind as she sailed down the hall.

"Dee," she gasped in panic, forgetting to address her properly as "Miss Rennie." "The electricity is out. The iron lungs. We have to rock them so they will keep working." With that, she turned and ran, and Dee charged behind her, quickly catching up.

They entered the ward where children stricken with polio lay, wrapped in their iron lungs, the metal cylinders that kept them alive. Known as tank ventilators, iron lungs helped people breathe who were stricken with polio. Without power, the iron lungs couldn't oscillate and help the children breathe. The children's faces were peeping out of the cylinders, and they clucked their tongues as Dee ran in—the only sign they could make to indicate they couldn't breathe. "Cluck-cluck-cluck" rang out in unison, their faces filled with apprehension. Dee grabbed one and Sister grabbed another.

A fellow student, Marcy, ran in; fortunately, between the three of them, they were able to rock the three patients and keep the iron lungs moving. Dee glanced over at Marcy—the student who consistently chewed in class. There was Marcy, rocking and chewing—whatever was in her mouth was giving her perfect rhythm. Dee almost felt a giggle bubble up; she knew it wasn't humor, but almost hysteria that was overwhelming her.

Dee could feel beads of sweat on her forehead. Her heart seemed to beat faster. Some more sisters and doctors came running to provide support and help keep the iron lungs going until the electricity turned back. When the humming came on and the lights flickered again, Dee almost dropped in relief. Mercifully, it was over.

Dee stroked a little girl's hair that peeped out of the iron lung. She could tell the girl had no fever. She knew Sister would come by to check each small patient thoroughly and the subsequent charting would be done. With tears in her eyes, Dee walked out of the ward, her steps heavy. Sick children were not for her, she told herself.

OBSTETRICS

The dreaded obstetrics shift was finally unavoidable. The student nurses worked split night shift, from 7 p.m. to 11 pm. and then 4 a.m. to 7 a.m. The students became experts at racing to the Nurses' Home to hop in their beds for roughly a four-hour sleep, by the time they undressed and got dressed again. Once on duty, the nuns greeted them with ghastly bologna and pickle sandwiches to help "wake them up." Dee wasn't sure what was worse—having her sleep interrupted or being made to eat something that would surely have brought her mother up to the hospital to bring her home forcibly if she knew what the nuns were feeding her darling daughter.

Dee soon learned, though, that being alert was important. Inarose, the redheaded victim of the fabled shower practical joke, had recently been involved in an incident long discussed by the students. Inarose had been working in the nursery formula kitchen. One jar of the powdered formula didn't look right, and she was told to throw it down the incinerator by the nun in charge. Shaking the contents of the jar into the incinerator, Inarose closed it and realized only half of the formula had gone down. Inarose opened the door to throw the rest down; the formula somehow reacted with the incinerator, igniting and blowing back up, throwing her across the room. One of her classmates came running, yelling, "Something's burning! Oh, it's Inarose," she added, stating the obvious.

Inarose was taken to Emergency, where she was covered with Butesin Picrate, a bright yellow ointment, and then covered with a gauze mask with holes for the eyes. Those who visited her quickly averted their eyes, wincing in pain. "That doesn't bode well for her love life," whispered some of her classmates as they exited Inarose's room. As always, the nursing students preferred to stick to the facts.

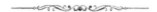

DEE YAWNED AS SHE WALKED AROUND THE NURSERY, adjusting the sleeping babies' blankets and laying a cool hand to their faces. Dee loved babies, but when they were all asleep, things got boring and she'd realize how sleepy she was.

The nights stretched on, many times with just Dee and her friend Sybil tending to the babies, who were all kept in the nursery rather than in the mothers' rooms. In the 1940s, mothers were often kept in the hospital for up to two weeks after giving birth. Dee preferred the babies over the tiresome mothers, who were hormonal and needed a lot of extra compassion after giving birth.

The nursery was a calm place to work, with Sister coming in and out occasionally, charting and checking on things.

As a baby woke up for a feeding, Dee went over to grab a glass bottle from the dresser, where Sybil had thoughtfully placed it in anticipation. Dee went to feed and rock the little girl back to sleep. All that rocking made her even more tired.

"Dee, you're practically asleep," whispered Sybil accusingly as she came in with another bottle. "Don't drop the baby!"

"I know. I know," grumbled Dee with a yawn.

As she put the now-sleeping baby back in her crib, she

glanced over and saw an empty iron crib. Since there were only a few babies in the nursery that night, things were a little slow.

Gesturing toward the crib, she told Sybil her idea: one of them could take a brief nap and the other could watch for Sister. Then they would trade. It sounded like a brilliant idea.

It *was* a brilliant idea, thought Dee contently, curled up in the large crib, which was perfect for someone of her size. She slept just like a baby, frowning when Sybil shook her roughly. As she sat up slowly, Dee heard Sister's rosary beads rattling as she walked with determination down the hall toward the nursery to check on her new charges.

Rubbing her eyes, Dee climbed out of the crib quickly, just in time to see Sister walk through the door. She narrowed her eyes at Dee, her mouth thin.

Dee and Sybil trudged back to the Nurses' Home after their shift that morning, walked in and paused at the switchboard. Remarkably, there was no note by Frances Rodgers. With a grin, Dee went to bed—again.

PSYCHIATRIC NURSING

Dee continued her rotations, including urological and orthopedics. It was now time for psychiatric nursing. After hearing stories from her friends, Dee traveled down to Salem for psychiatric nursing with a heavy heart. Because Salem was about 45 miles south of Portland, the student nurses stayed in dormitories for three months while they worked at the Oregon State Mental Hospital. Their syllabus described lectures and clinical demonstration of various psychoses, stressing the etiology, mental mechanics, symptomology, diagnoses, treatment, nursing care, and prevention of functional and organic mental diseases.

Unofficially, Dee had heard the whispers about how this

would be the hardest rotation. She knew in her heart it would be.

The state hospital, a large cavernous and gloomy building, was as scary and intimidating as nursing could be. There were stories of it being haunted, and Dee believed it, shivering and staying close to her friends as they ran to work. They saw operations and heard stories about techniques used on patients that seemed barbaric.

The one thing the students were taught was never forget to count the needles, sharps and knives used for any procedure before, during and after. Dee was meticulous about this, often writing it down to ensure she had the proper count, shuddering at the thought if she didn't.

On some days the nursing students turned on music, though, and the patients stood shakily, swayed and smiled. Music seemed to soothe and bring joy to the often-gloomy unit. The nursing students would dance with some of the patients and, for a moment, life seemed more positive and filled with light.

After those three months, the girls were finished and allowed to travel back to St. Vincent. They talked little about their experiences there, and they all vowed that it took a special someone to consider psychiatric nursing for these vulnerable human beings. Dee knew someone had to do it, but it wasn't going to be her.

"I'm going to be a surgical nurse," she told herself with resolve.

THE GRAVITY OF WAR

I t was 1944, and the world was still at war. Dee worried constantly about her cousins—their letters were few and far between, and she had no idea where any of them were. She looked at the framed pictures of each of them on her desk, saying a quick Hail Mary every day for their safety.

The war deeply affected all supplies and daily life. The nurses still had trouble buying their hose, getting adept at stitching holes together when they were forced to. The students would stay up at nights, often grouped in a room together, making little pill cups out of random scraps of paper. Wartime meant that every single item must be reviewed for its ability to be recycled. Almost all of the surgical dressings, gauze hot packs, swabs, perineal pads, cotton applicators, cotton and pill cups were made by nurses or nursing students convalescing from brief illnesses or when they had spare time. Even surgical and obstetrics' rubber gloves were washed, dried and mended to be reused. Rubber bands were made out of rubber gloves that could no longer be used. Empty alcohol bottles were filled with hot water to warm the post-op beds. The Sisters of Providence were adept at the recycling business.

Few people in the city traveled anywhere because tires were threadbare and there was no gasoline to spare. Food was rationed and the shelves at most local stores were constantly depleted. The world was a dark, scary place; Dee would often wonder if the war was ever going to end. She watched students graduate, quickly leaving to join the Army Nurse Corps and travel where they were needed as part of the war effort. Fear gripped her at times, making the weight of these years almost unbearable. It was only the hard work, learning new things and the short bursts of joy with her friends at the Nurses' Home that saw her through this difficult time.

Dee was charting one night, the ward quiet around her. She loved this time of night, when most patients had been washed, tucked in and were sleeping soundly. Getting them to bed was no simple task. The patients had to be lifted often and adjusted in their beds to ensure they were positioned appropriately. Dee felt compassion for the patients who needed lots of back rubs to ease pain. She knew it was hard to get comfortable, especially in the hospital's narrow, old-fashioned iron beds. Dee routinely went to whichever sister was on duty to beg for more pillows to tuck around the patients. Each sister assigned to a floor was in charge of doling out linens, and often it took a little persuasion to get certain nuns to release an extra pillow or blanket. The nuns were conscious of the extra workload this made for the laundry department, as well as the extra soap and water it took.

On this particular night, though, everyone peacefully slept and Dee was thankful she didn't have to take any vitals for a few hours, allowing her to catch up on her notes. Ozzy demanded that the nursing students chart throughout their shifts, as was required of nurses. Dee, always trying to make sure her patients were comfortable, often got sidetracked with an extra sponge bath or running to the kitchen and pleading with Sister Cresence for some pudding or toast for a hungry patient.

Dee's charting method was to write on medicine cards—scraps of paper she stuck in her pockets. By dinner, those pockets were bulging, and she pushed them down further as Ozzy inevitably walked by, suspiciously eyeing the lumps in Dee's pockets.

Dee carefully transferred her notes to the patients' charts in the chart room. Trying to decipher her writing, she was holding a scrap up with a furrowed brow when Sister Bertina came running through the hall. Out of breath, she stopped in the doorway, unable to speak.

"Sister, what's wrong?" Dee cried.

"The curtains, Dee," she gasped finally. "Get the curtains."

"Oh God," Dee thought, "Not again."

Annabelle ran toward Dee from the dark hall, her face flushed, her hair falling down from its pins. Together, the students ran into the wards, pulling down the blackout curtains quickly and shutting off any lamps that had been left on. They heard the air raid sirens in the distance, blaring through the once-still night, and they each felt adrenaline and fear coursing through their veins.

"What's going on?" asked some of the men sleepily, sitting up in the larger of the wards that contained nine beds. Some simply muttered, "Again?" and turned over.

"Air drill," Dee whispered, trying to appear calmer than she felt. One of these times, she feared it would not be a drill. The hospital blacked out as much as they could during these drills, the lights off, the black curtains in place. The brick fortress sat silently in the night, a dark shadow against the nearby hill.

After racing around and taking one more lap to peer into each room, Dee silently tread down the hall, returning to the now-dark chart room. Annabelle soon joined her, slumping into a chair. The two stared at each other in the darkened room, both uneasy. There was nothing to do now, as Dee wasn't motivated to finish her charting by flashlight. Fortunately, it wasn't long before Sister came back, turning on the light above their heads. The drill was over. The shades would come up in the morning, rather than disturb patients by doing it now. All was fine, but Dee still felt queasy—it never seemed to get easier. Her shoulders felt very heavy.

Recently, everyone had read about D-Day, and Dee saw the headlines in papers that patients shared with her. The battle, which began on June 6, 1944, included 156,000 American, British and Canadian forces landing on five beaches along a 50-mile stretch of the heavily fortified coast of France's Normandy region. The invasion was one of the largest military assaults of the war, and Dee and her friends discussed it constantly. Many of the students nervously wondered if their relatives or boyfriends were involved, since it was reported to be such a large invasion. They also heard thousands were killed or injured. News was filtering out from the war in bits and pieces, leaving all the girls wondering about their loved ones.

Though Dee was anxious for news of her cousins, she was forced to put it out of her mind at work. Often, she would quietly ask her mother if there was any news from Theresa's sister, Dorothy. Though her Aunt Dorothy was always cheerful, Dee knew Nini and Fef's safety weighed heavily on her. Dee didn't want to add to her burden by bringing it up.

That morning following the drill, Dee quietly lifted the shades, peering out at her beloved Mount Hood. Bare now in the summer with just a little white on top, it sat in contrast to the blue sky.

It was a beautiful summer day, and Dee soaked it in for a minute, thinking how the brightness of the day was a stark contrast to the fearful night. She yawned as she finished putting up the shades, whispering to her friends as they came on duty. It had been a quiet night despite the air drill, and there wasn't much to report.

Dee hurried to the Nurses' Home, thinking about her bed. She pulled open the great door, looking automatically to see if there was a message for her at the switchboard. She glanced at the notes near Frances Rodgers, but there were none for her.

"Dee?"

Dee pivoted quickly to see her father standing in the front parlor. Just a few inches taller than her, today he looked smaller, his face ashen.

Dee's heart pounded. She could barely move her mouth to form the words she desperately needed to ask.

"Oh, Dad, which one?" she finally whispered.

"Nini. Normandy."

And Dee sobbed as her heart broke.

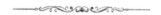

THE FAMILY HAD RECEIVED WORD THAT STAFF SERGEANT Anthony Rennie, Company A, 1st Battalion 22nd Infantry, 4th Infantry Division, was killed in France, in the Saint-Lô area during Operation Cobra, an offensive after the Normandy campaign on July 27, 1944—almost exactly one year from when he entered the Army. He was just 19.

Dee said later she was surprised when her father told her it was Nini who had perished. Nini, who barely stood 5-foot-6, seemed larger than life, with his constant laughter and enthusiastic embrace of life. For some reason, Dee always thought it would be Fef. Fef had always stood by her side like a sentinel, and Dee knew he would do the same for his fellow soldiers, undoubtedly putting himself in harm's way. Either way, Dee was heartbroken that she had lost one of her dearest cousins and friends.

Soon after, the family received a letter from Fef. He reassured them he would be coming home—that even the United States Army would not rob his mother of another son.

There was no funeral. Dee went home and comforted her family, but without a body, Father Troy, their parish priest, said a funeral could not be held. The family went to St. Philip Neri and prayed anyway.

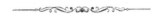

TIME PASSED WITH MORE AIR DRILLS, MORE RATIONING AND dark days. The news sounded encouraging, though, and the students were hopeful the war was ending. Many of the student nurses had boyfriends (or even secret husbands) who were still alive, and the hope was that if the war would end, the darkness would lift and life as they knew it would return.

It was the summer of 1945, and Dee was riding the streetcar with Annabelle. The old streetcars in Portland rumbled from the base of Northwest 23rd near the hospital all the way across town. Dee and Annabelle were on their way to Providence on the city's East Side to hear a pediatric lecture from a visiting physician.

They talked quietly on the streetcar. Too hot for their blue capes, Dee and Annabelle stood out in their starched white nurses' uniforms. Suddenly the street car operator brought the car to a resounding halt on the edge of the city's downtown core. The women grabbed on to each other, almost landing on the streetcar's floor.

"What in the world?" Dee wondered out loud. The girls then glanced outside. People began running from shops and businesses. Men and women shouted, crossing the streetcar line and blocking it from inching down the street. Everyone outside was dancing and singing. It was a kaleidoscope of colors as if, in slow motion, the world was coming out of its darkness to celebrate.

The war was over.

Portland's Mayor Earl Riley immediately ordered all the liquor stores and nightclubs closed on August 14, 1945, the fateful day that Japan surrendered. He hoped to maintain order, but it was beyond his control. The party downtown lasted for days.

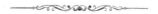

SOON AFTER, DEE'S BELOVED FEF APPEARED. HE GRABBED Dee and swung her around and around, hugging her tightly.

"How in the world did you get here so fast?" she laughed. Simple, he told her. He was on the train, headed up to Fort Lewis in Washington to be processed and decommissioned. When he saw the signs for Portland, Fef simply jumped off. "Why go all the way up to Fort Lewis to come right back down again?" he said with his usual shrug and practical smile.

Dee was beyond happy to see him. She talked to her friends about her cousin coming home, even bringing some of them home with her for a big family dinner.

Over a meal of spaghetti and meatballs, Fef, who should have been excited about eating his mother's and aunt's home cooking, seemed distracted. Dee glanced across the table at one of her classmates who had come home with her, Polly Krueger, and then back to Fef and smiled. Polly, with black curls and a big wide smile, was a year younger than Dee. Dee hadn't thought about any of her friends becoming romantic with her cousin, but she saw instantly their connection.

Now that the men were coming home, there were dances and pop-up baseball games on the hill up and beyond the hospital. Dee was happy to have her dancing partner home again and invited Fef to the dances. As she watched him whirling Polly around the dance floor, Dee knew then she had lost her other dance partner. The couple was later married in 1947 after Polly graduated. They eventually raised eight children in Northeast Portland and celebrated 50 years of marriage. Fef always saved a dance for Dee, though.

A few years after Nini's death, his mother, Dorothy, discovered that his remains had been buried in France. She paid a significant amount of money to fly her son home. "You don't even know if that's him in that casket," sniffed the ever-practical Theresa. Dorothy determinedly did it anyway, finally able to have a funeral at St. Philip Neri. She buried Nini beside his father, Pete, on a gentle slope at Mount Calvary Cemetery on Portland's West Side, because she said it was the right thing to do.

A NEW CHAPTER

Graduation was here! After taking 216 credits and completing countless rotations, Dee and the rest of the other 38 survivors from the Class of 1946 were graduating. Dee couldn't believe the day had finally arrived, but she had mixed feelings. Graduating meant finally achieving her goal of being a nurse, yet it also brought an end to all the fun and closeness she had felt on her little hill. Dee would miss her friends desperately. Some were staying, many were getting married and moving on, and several were still joining the Army Nurses Corps, which now that the war was over, promised travel and adventure.

The nurses would be honored at ceremonies at both the St. Vincent School of Nursing and then one with the entire student body at the University of Portland. The first ceremony involved receiving their St. Vincent School of Nursing pins. Dee stood in line with her classmates and, after receiving a corsage, held still as Sister Genevieve gently affixed the small STV pin to her uniform.

All the graduating nurses had professional photos taken in their black gowns and mortar boards as well as in their nurses' uniforms. Thanks to the camera's filter that blurred her face around the edges, Dee's looked especially glamorous, as if she was a movie star with her deep lipstick and wavy black, shoulder-length hair. The photographer had captured the gaze in her brown eyes: a look of quiet strength and determination, as well as a lot of pride.

The night before the first graduation, the girls gathered upstairs in the Nurses' Home. Clad in their usual pajamas, robes and with rollers in their hair, they drank champagne and laughed at their antics. "Remember Dee's bed in the elevator?" they laughed. "Remember the Peeping Tom on the fire escape?" they shrieked. They laughed, remembering the beer they had snuck in, throwing the bottles in the shrubbery behind the Nurses' Home before Tillie, the housemother, came to do bed check. Tense days followed when the gardeners came, and a student nurse was dispatched to keep Sister occupied while the gardeners filled a garbage sack with the empty, discarded bottles. The students giggled, remembering how the gardeners would shake their heads, but never rat them out.

The soon-to-be graduates remembered the late-night raids of ice cream in the hospital's basement, the trips to Henry Thiele's to sit in the back room, the quiet nights gathered in their rooms, sharing their dreams in whispers and with careful hope. They reminisced about their ragtag baseball games behind the hospital and the basketball games on the court in the Nurses' Home. One by one, they gave toasts, from the most gregarious to the quietest among them. Even Miss Encyclopedia of the World stood up. A little tipsy now, she reminisced about her favorite classes and didn't correct anybody once. The Class of 1946 toasted Ozzy, their mentor, who despite terrifying them, was direct and fair, and shaped them into excellent nurses. And then they cried and vowed that they would be bonded through life—almost as true sisters.

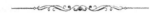

THE ST. VINCENT SCHOOL OF NURSING GRADUATION WAS held in the auditorium at the Nursing School. Ozzy, Sister Genevieve, Father John and many of the priests, doctors and nuns sat on the dais, smiling like proud parents. Dee watched her friends, one by one, receive their diplomas. There went Dorothy, Shirley, Rosemary, and dear Sybil, waving to her family as she walked across the stage. MaryAnn, class president, made a small speech and beamed. Annabelle almost danced across the stage in her inimitable fashion.

Finally, it was Rose Marie Rennie's turn—although no one ever really knew her by that name. In fact, most frequently, she was called by her maiden name, Rennie or Little Rennie by her classmates—almost as an endearment. Dee received her diploma, shook hands and turned to face the crowd. She saw her parents right away, as if there was a small spotlight on them. Her mother was clapping enthusiastically, and her father beamed—his grin couldn't get any bigger. Dee stood for a minute, savoring their parental pride. Gone were the days of her parents' apprehension regarding her decision to be a nurse; they were united in their love for her and couldn't be prouder.

The stress wasn't over, though. The graduates now faced taking the dreaded state nursing exam. They studied for weeks, which Dee found overwhelming at times. They took the hours-long test, walking out with mixed feelings on how well they did. When the envelopes arrived in late summer, Dee and her friends gathered together, holding the still-sealed envelopes nervously.

"You open mine," Dee thrust hers at Annabelle. With a

lot of arguing and back and forth, they finally ripped into them. They all shrieked in happiness when they realized they all passed; Ozzy would have expected nothing less of them.

Fortunately, Dee knew she had a job already. She had been summoned to Ozzy's office prior to graduation to discuss her aspirations. Dee told Ozzy what she had been thinking about for some time; she loved the Operating Room. "I'd really like to be a surgical nurse," she said, her head in the clouds, thinking about how much she enjoyed witnessing all the surgeons' new techniques and specialized skills.

Ozzy just looked at her thoughtfully, and Dee had a bad feeling in the pit of her stomach. Finally, Ozzy commanded, "Miss Rennie, you are too good with the patients to be in surgery. You'll work 2 North."

Dee opened her mouth to argue, but after one look at Ozzy, and she knew the decision was final.

Those words rang in her head as Dee began her nursing career at 2 North. It was the toughest department, and she knew it. She watched the student nurses come in, hardly believing she had ever been that inexperienced. She took pity on them, though, showing them everything she knew. Dee lived at home and commuted by streetcar from the family's home, still in Ladd's Addition. She loved her job, even though the days were long and the work was hard.

One day as Dee got off work, she found her father waiting for her in the hospital's lobby, standing erect, holding his fedora in his hands. At first, she was alarmed, thinking back to the last time he waited for her after her shift. "Dad, what's wrong?" she asked frantically. Frank smiled, his big grin lighting up his face, and Dee knew he wasn't there to deliver any bad news.

"Come on, Dee," he said simply. When Dee pulled up hours later in front of their house in her brand-new 1946 midnight blue Chevrolet, Theresa just shook her head, but her big smile revealed to Dee that her parents had made this decision together.

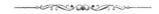

Unfortunately, one of Dee's first outings with her new Chevrolet wasn't a positive one. Getting off duty from 2 North late as usual, she was hurrying to get to the bank to cash her small paycheck. Finally locating a meter on a downtown corner, she plugged it with the first coin she could find and tore into the bank, her short legs flying. There was a longer line in the bank than she anticipated; when she finally emerged, she walked to the corner to retrieve her car. She looked up from her deposit slip she had been studying to see an officer standing near her precious car, writing a parking ticket.

"Officer," she shouted, running ahead. "There was a long line at the bank and I put money in the meter. I'm here now so I can just drive it away."

The officer looked at her with his eyebrows raised, taking in her nurse's uniform and her anxious face. At first Dee thought she had swayed him until he ripped off the ticket, placing it with a clap on her windshield.

Dee's eyebrows snapped together, and her lips drew into a frown. She was a polite person and not one to wish others ill will, but she was furious that this officer would not consider her plight.

Grabbing the ticket and looking at the hefty fine, she said the first thing to come to mind:

"I hope you have to have gallbladder surgery someday!"

Satisfied, she smiled and drove away, knowing that at the time gallbladder surgery was one of the absolute worst surgeries to recover from. She tried not to look in her rearview mirror at the officer, who was now standing in the street, scratching his head.

THAT MIDNIGHT BLUE CHEVY SOON BECAME FAMOUS around the University of Portland campus, especially since few young people had new cars. Since the men were back from war, it meant the women, even those who had graduated, were now hanging around the University of Portland campus.

Going out to the Bluff was a regular occurrence for Dee and her friends. The only problem was that Dee couldn't parallel park, and parking was limited. She and her friends would often circle the campus several times, looking for the premium corner space for the big car. "We'll be around again," Sybil would shout as she leaned out the car, her blonde wavy hair flying, her cat-eye glasses shining, as she waved at cute guys.

The return of males to the campus also meant football was back, and the University of Portland had cobbled together a football team, as did most of the local colleges. One day, Dee and her friends decided to drive down to watch a game at Oregon State University, about 85 miles south of Portland. Having one of the few cars around the college meant that word spread among students about an opportunity to get a ride to the game. Dee and her friends were waiting at her house for Sybil to arrive when two guys appeared at her door. One carried a bag of apples, and both of them chewed on an apple as they blended in with the group. The interlopers seemed to know the rest of the guys present, but Dee had never seen them before.

One of the two was Ed Wallo, a tall, broad-chested, handsome man with a head of beautiful dark hair, bright blue eyes and a dimpled chin. Hailing from Pennsylvania, he had been stationed in Santa Barbara while in the Marines, where he taught bayonet fighting, judo and combat swimming. He longed to see action, but the Marines found him far more valuable as an instructor, with his strong physique and quick agility.

Ed had soon met Sam Cavalli on the base. Sam, gregarious and a natural dealmaker, was from Portland. He promptly promised Ed and a band of guys from the East Coast that if they came to Portland after the war, he'd secure them all football scholarships at the University of Portland. They showed up and remarkably, Sam made good on his promise. He twisted the arms of the Holy Cross priests who were eager to build the university into a thriving institution. The priests knew from their experience at Notre Dame that football was the way to college prosperity.

When confident, handsome, extroverted Ed Wallo walked into a room, people knew it. He talked to anyone who would listen, his dry wit always prevalent. His sidekick was Tony Koreiva. Smaller than Ed, and definitely much quieter, Tony came from a close-knit Lithuanian family from Chicago. He had amiable manners, a great sense of humor and he knew how to be Ed's straight man, laughing at all his jokes and setting him up for more. The two were assigned to be roommates when they first arrived and had become fast friends.

Ed and Tony heard about a girl who had a new car and was going to drive to the game; it was Ed's idea to find their way to her house, turn on the charm and hitch a ride. They underestimated Dee, however, and completely overplayed their hand.

Dee sized them up instantly. Two rude easterners, she sniffed, watching them eat their apples and not offer any to the group. When the bigger one complained they would miss kickoff because of Sybil's tardiness, Dee showed them the door. "Get out of my house," she said, "and don't come back," she added, as she closed the door with a final slam.

A few months later, Dee went to a dance at the University of Portland. Dressed up and looking gorgeous, she easily had many partners. Soon she found herself dancing with one Ed Wallo, who she found breathtakingly handsome. She did not associate him with the football encounter, the apples or his rudeness. She had heard about him, though. He was the talk of the campus, and many women had been plotting to set their caps for him.

Dee was no stranger to popularity. She had already turned down a few beaus who had proposed. She said no for the sole reason that she had not fallen in love with any of her suitors. She smugly thought that she'd hook the elusive Ed Wallo just to show that she could and later dump him when she was no longer interested. The two began dating and soon after spotting the midnight blue Chevrolet, Ed put two and two together and sheepishly confessed they had met before. Dee wasn't swayed by the memory; however, and the two continued dating.

Just nine months after the dance, Ed asked Dee to marry him. Unfortunately, his prospects didn't look too good on paper. Even with the football scholarship, Ed badly needed money and desperately wanted to finish his education. He knew how he could make some quick cash. Prior to joining the Marines, Ed had been a professional boxer. Starting early in his youth, he grabbed the identification of his older brother, Michael, and began boxing in amateur fights. When he became old enough, he used his own identification and adopted the name of "Rocco Wallo," fighting in more than 100 amateur matches. As an amateur, he won the British Gloves Champion trophy in 1941.

Turning pro, Ed continued, but then the war hit. That didn't deter his boxing ability; he ending up winning the 1944

Championship of the West Coast United States Marine Corps Stations' 180-pound league.

Now Ed's best moneymaking prospect was to go back to boxing, but he didn't want to leave Dee. "Marry me," he said. "But we have to leave right after Christmas because I have a fight on New Year's Eve. I have to go with or without you."

Despite the practical, unromantic proposal, Dee wanted to be with him. She was very much in love with Ed, but she needed more time. She quickly realized her parents would not be thrilled at the prospect of their only child taking off for the East Coast with a man they barely knew, so she hatched a plan: "We have to be married in the church," she told him. Ed, also a devout Catholic, readily agreed. Dee assumed Father Troy, who had known her for years, would balk at marrying the couple in just a couple weeks. After all, this was all going too fast. She figured after the priest's refusal, Ed could go back East, set up some fights, make some money and return to Portland. They would have a big wedding and settle in Portland, she mused to herself.

"I trust your judgment, Dee," Father Troy said at the end of his interview with the couple, hugging Dee and clapping Ed on the back. The couple had gone in timorously, but Ed had taken over, using his charm and talking to the priest as if he had known him for a lifetime. Ed had a way with priests, having already made friends with several of them at the University of Portland, including the Dutch Masters.

Ed easily convinced Father Troy that this match meant to be. The couple was married in a small ceremony on December 27, 1947. Because it was Christmas break, their closest friends were home in other cities with their families and could not be there. Theresa and Frank swallowed hard as they watched the newlyweds drive off in the midnight blue Chevrolet on their long drive to the East Coast. Dee gazed out the back window until they were out of sight. She gave

Ed a tremulous smile, but deep inside, a slight tug of her heart gave her pause.

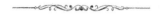

DEE WAS NERVOUS. HER JOB INTERVIEW WAS WITH THE matron of a hospital in Orange, New Jersey. The hospital was close to Ed's immediate family, who had resettled in New Jersey. The couple had very little money, and Dee knew she needed a solid job while Ed looked for boxing matches in New York.

Sitting on the hard chair, Dee tried not to squirm, twisting her wedding ring—delicate with just a few precious small diamonds—around and around on her small finger. The matron sat behind her wooden desk, facing Dee. It was not a Catholic hospital and there was not a nun in sight, which felt odd to Dee who had grown accustomed to having the sisters around every corner. Dee was anxious as she watched the matron read her application, double checking things, turning pages slowly.

Suddenly, she glanced up over her glasses, looking at Dee inquisitively.

"I see you're one of Ozzy's girls," she smiled, putting her fountain pen down and sitting back in her chair. "That means you must be good."

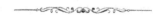

DEE AND ED'S TIME IN NEW JERSEY WAS A FRESH beginning, but it also held struggle. The couple, very much in love, found settling into a new routine difficult. Though it was home for Ed, Dee felt like she was on foreign soil. Ed's parents and two sisters and two brothers were caring, hard-working people. However, this East Coast family differed greatly from her family in so many ways. Ed's father, Michael, had lost his wife, Julia, at an early age, shortly after she gave birth to their third child, a baby girl. Ed and his older brother, Mike, were sent to an orphanage as their devastated father headed back to his job in the coal mines. Julia's young sister, Helen, took care of the newborn baby, Delores— lovingly nicknamed Dolly. After a time, it came as no surprise that Helen, just 21 years old, stepped up and married the now 36-year-old Michael—an act of selflessness that was probably assumed to be her duty. The boys were then brought home from the orphanage, and the couple had two more children. Ed worshipped his new mother, realizing that because of her, he and his brother were now able to return home.

Ed's father, "Pop," as the family referred to him, was a complex man. He was kind and generous soul, a devout Catholic, and had built a life for himself with very little education. He had many professions over the years, working as a coal miner, painter and police officer. He had a sensitive side, writing stories, songs and poetry for his own enjoyment. The sensitive side seemed to disappear quickly, though; he was also loud, deeply opinionated and eccentric, yelling expletives out the window at the neighbors they shared a driveway with. Pop and the neighbors were in constant battle over parking spots, garbage cans, and other daily compromises. No one seemed to bat an eye when he would spring from the table in the middle of a meal, yank open the window and call the neighbor all sorts of names Dee had never even heard until now.

Worse for Dee, meals were over quickly—the family sat down, ate quickly and left the table with Dee just half finished with her meal. Dee sighed as she reminisced about her Italian family, lingering over cheese, nuts and wine, discussing all the latest events in a leisurely fashion.

Ed and Dee first moved in with their in-laws, taking turns

sleeping on a twin bed—the other in a chair. Realizing that was not a long-term situation as newlyweds, they soon looked for a place to live. They landed at a boarding house, renting a small room from a woman, who also habitually screamed at the neighbors. Dee began to see this behavior as normal.

Ed was gone a lot, working with his manager, Jack Toner, to get signed on to as many boxing matches as he could in New York. Ed appeared in boxing matches frequently at Madison Square Garden and spent his days practicing. Known for his right jab, he spent hours perfecting it with his large hands and quick reflexes.

Dee went once with Ed's sister Dolly to watch him box. Grown up now, Dolly was just a few years younger than Dee, and was a striking blonde with a big smile. She and Dee made a statement when they walked in the room together. Settling into their seats at the boxing match, Dee soon realized attending was a mistake. Though Ed was a strong, agile, light heavyweight fighter, she watched him become bruised and battered. Dolly, oblivious to Dee's horror, joined others in shouting encouragement in the form of beating his opponent to a pulp. After it was over, Ed had won in a knockout, but a shattered Dee grabbed Dolly and the two quickly left. Dee promised herself she would never watch Ed box again. She made good on that vow.

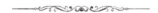

DEE SETTLED INTO A ROUTINE, WORKING LONG SHIFTS AT the hospital in Orange, and then routinely stopped at her in-laws on the way home to have a beer with her mother-in-law. Helen provided a little companionship and looked forward to this habit now with her new daughter-in-law. Dee frequently waved off the cabbage dinners the Slovakian woman was always cooking, instead going home to her one-room studio, thinking longingly of her mother's Italian cooking.

To pass the time, Dee taught Ed's younger brother, Earle, how to drive and befriended his much younger sister, Bernadene, who was only 9. When Ed was home, they went dancing or out to dinner with his older brother, Mike, and his new bride, Clara. Ed and Dee found a comfortable friendship with the unassuming couple, who were also very much in love and had met during the war when Mike had been stationed in the south. A true Southern belle, gentle and kind to the core, Clara hailed from Pascagoula, Mississippi, and also felt a little out of place. The two women soon formed a lifelong kinship.

Dee tried to make the best of it, but she lost weight, getting down to just 99 pounds; she was so homesick, she could barely stand it. While she loved Ed's family, life on the East Coast was unfamiliar, very rushed, and most of all, she missed her family, friends and the comfortable familiarity of her city. She found the new hospital cold and sterile, and she missed St. Vincent Hospital, the warmth and care of the Sisters of Providence and all her friends there.

One day, Ed came back to their small studio. He had a look of determination on his face and quietly said, "Let's go home."

"Where's home?" Dee asked, her heart beating wildly, afraid to even hope for what she was hearing. "Portland," he answered. Dee recalled later her bags were packed and put in the midnight blue Chevrolet as if she was evacuating for a hurricane.

After a brief stop in Washington, D.C., to see Dee's cousin Bud and his wife, Francis, the couple returned to Portland. Ed told her on the way home he longed for Oregon again. He loved the slower pace, the beauty of the mountains contrasting with the rugged coastline. He called it "God's

Country," and though he would miss his family, he couldn't wait to get back to his newly adopted home.

Dee's parents were thrilled and eager to assist the couple in settling back in. Frank owned a small row of brick apartments in Northeast Portland, and Dee and Ed moved in, surrounded by other couples their age.

Ed went back to school at the University of Portland. He valued higher education and wanted to become an English teacher and possibly a football coach.

Dee found herself back in Ozzy's office, asking for a job. She prayed Ozzy would be merciful.

"2 North, Mrs. Wallo," said Ozzy.

"I thought I could possibly go to surgery ..." Dee trailed off as Ozzy raised her eyebrows.

"2 North," Ozzy insisted. "You're the only one who can handle it, Dee," she finally admitted quietly, with a small apologetic smile.

Dee smiled and shrugged. It didn't matter. She was home.

PHOTOS

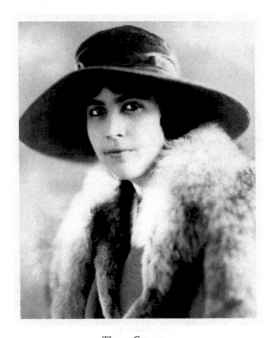

Theresa Greco, 1919

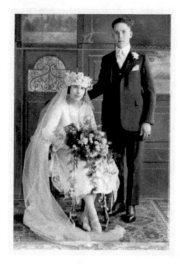

Frank and Theresa Rennie Wedding Day, 1922

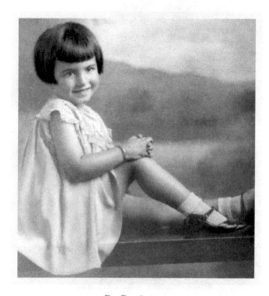

Dee Rennie, 1929

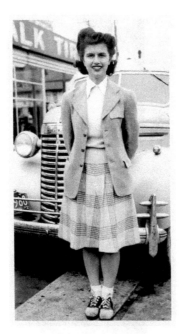

Dee Rennie poses while in high school, 1940

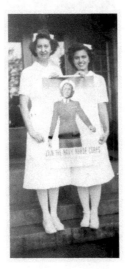

*Dee and Pat in front of Nurses' Home helping recruit nurses for
the Army Corps*

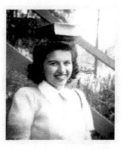

Dee shows a special skill

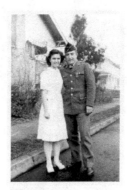

Dee and Nini spend time together before he ships out for the Army

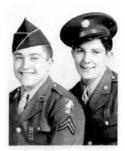

The two brothers, Nini (left) and John (Fef) pose in their military uniforms during WWII

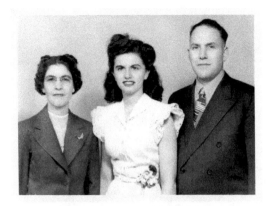

Dee and her parents, Frank and Theresa, 1946

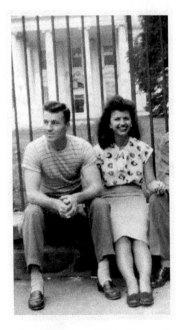

Dee and Ed in front of White House, 1948

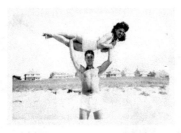

Ed shows his special skills on the beach in Seaside, Oregon, 1947

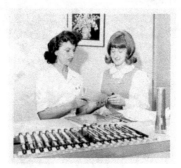

Dee teaches a candy striper what to do on 2 North in 1966
(Photo courtesy Providence Archives, Seattle)

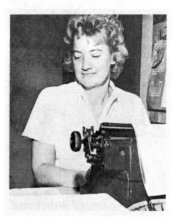

Mary Schmidt, Unit Secretary on 2 North, 1966 (Photo courtesy
Providence Archives, Seattle)

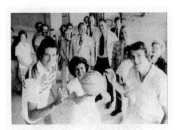

Dee with Trail Blazers Bob Gross (left) and Geoff Petrie (right) kick off the 9th Floor renovation (Photo courtesy Providence Archives, Seattle)

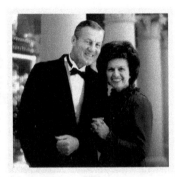

Dee and Ed, 1983

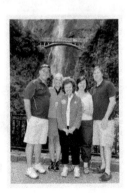

Dee with children (from left) Steve, MaryJo, Terri and Edward at Multnomah Falls

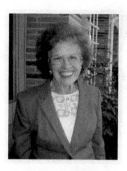

Dee attends one of the last Homecomings

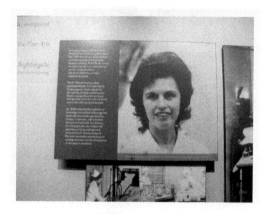

Dee's tribute wall hangs at St. Vincent Hospital on the 2nd floor

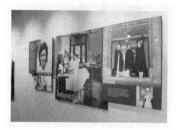

Dee's tribute wall is in the north hallway on the 2nd floor

PUBLISHED MONTHLY
BY THE STUDENTS OF
ST. VINCENT SCHOOL
OF NURSING

Sec. 435½, P. L. & R.
U. S. POSTAGE
1c Paid
Portland, Oregon
Permit No. 738

Vincentian

Vol. 1   PORTLAND, OREGON, AUGUST, 1931   No. 8

Hardships of Pioneer Days Told

Portland Nurse Crosses Columbia in Rowboat Amid Ice

By MARGARET A. TYNAN, R. N.

This is the eighth of a series of articles dealing with the history of St. Vincent School of Nursing.

FOLLOWING graduation, Miss McDowell continued private duty, and during thirteen years of active service this was mostly social work. Dr. Bombrake at Goldendale, Washington, called her often, not only for typhoid fever and pneumonia cases but also for surgical work. He always informed the family that the nurse had to face the busy time during the afternoons. If the case was in town and it was not possible for her to take her rest undisturbed at the patient's home, he had her go to his house.

Of the many trips that she made to Goldendale one in particular was interesting since it gives an a good picture of the hardships of early spring travel. To go to Goldendale in those days one took the train to Grants, Oregon, ferried across the Columbia and went from there by horse and buggy. When Miss McDowell reached Grants, she found that the ferry was not running because of the ice floes in the river. Instead of returning to Portland as the ferry man had suggested, she argued with him that she had to reach the Washington side because there was a very sick pneumonia patient at Goldendale. When he saw that he could not deter her from her purpose, he said that he might be able to find a man who would be willing to row her across, but he also added that only a fool would risk his life in that mass of ice. About an hour later she started across the river, and then she realized that the ferryman was right. The man had a hard time keeping the boat in its course, and in the middle of the river they almost upset. This really did frighten her, but it was only for an instant. The thought of George Washington crossing the Delaware *(Continued on Page 6)*

HARRIETT E. OSBORN

ANOTHER member of St. Vincent's Alumnae who has contributed greatly to the advancement of higher educational standards in the school of nursing is Miss Harriett E. Osborn, at present Director of Education at St. Vincent School of Nursing.

Miss Osborn was born in Dawson City, Yukon Territory, Canada. After finishing high school there she entered the University of Oregon. To quote the Oregonian of June 12, 1929, concerning St. Vincent School of Nursing and commencement exercises: "Peculiar interest attaches to this graduation because Harriett Edita Osborn, one of the class, is by far the first recipient of the degree of bachelor of arts from the University of Oregon course in nursing. The system of having the university and hospital work together in giving nursing work is a new one with Miss Osborn as the first graduate" in the First Year Nursing Course under the School of Applied Social Science. During her hospital training she was employed as superintendent of the nurses into a student body called St. Vincent Hospital School of Nursing Corporation of which she was the first presiding officer. Also, as a student, she was the freshman who involved Dr. Sabin's honorary scholarship.

In the fall of 1929 she returned to St. Vincent's as general instructor of nurses. In developing a plan of the correlation of theory and practice in the school of nursing instruction were placed in the different departments of the hospital to instruct further the students in actual practice. Later followed the introduction of the preceptor grading system, and the systematized procedures in the wards.

At this year's annual spring election of the Oregon State Graduate Nurses' Association Miss Osborn was elected State Treasurer.

For the many things she has already done, for the many more she stands ready to do, and for the fine example she sets for the professional woman, and real friend the students take this opportunity to express their gratitude and appreciation to Miss Osborn.

5-Year Nursing Students Organize at University

THE five-year nursing students of Multnomah and St. Vincent's have recently organized into a Portland chapter of the Alpha Tau nursing sorority at the University at Eugene.

Alpha Tau was organized on the campus in the fall of 1927 and has been active since then in interesting girls to take advantage of the college education in connection with nurse's training. Because of the spirit shown in this group a well known national nursing honorary has taken an interest in the organization and definite plans for affiliation have been laid for the fall.

This Portland chapter which includes 18 to 20 girls from Eugene, and other campuses was definitely organized on August 10. At this meeting by-laws were drawn up and officers elected as follows:

President, Eva Davis; vice-president, Greta Shepard; secretary-treasurer, Catherine Pinkston; sergeant-at-arms, Charlotte Jamieson.

The first regular meeting of the organization will be held early in September.

Adopt Plan of Training for Internes

New System at St. Vincent's Went Into Effect on July First

By Dr. Hugh Brown

A PLAN for the training of the junior interne in a systematized manner made its appearance at St. Vincent's hospital on July 1 of this year. Despite the differences which appeared in the routine to which all it concerned with the hospital had been accustomed, despite the many changes in the activities of the internes, after some forty days, the plan seems to work and to prove the new curriculum have been upheld. Such a result is gratifying.

Co-operation has been excellent. The interns, the doctors, the graduates and the undergraduate nurses and all others connected with the hospital have considerably done their part in trying to allow this plan to succeed. Inasmuch as the success of these ideas is dependent upon such co-operation, we ask the continuance of the good will which has been shown. We appreciate that which has already been shown.

Briefly, to explain the purpose of the changes which have taken place: the board of governors, the interne committee, and the others of the hospital, wish to create at St. Vincent's hospital a period of training for young physicians which shall be second to none. In doing this their desires are many. The interne shall be given ample opportunity to display in actual work the result of a long period of training which for the most part has been in the abstract. He shall be given leeway in a certain degree in transposing his knowledge acquired as a practical basis, he will associate the ideas gathered and learned while at school to the practical aspect of practicing medicine. This interne must be aware, if the interne is to spend his time profitably for twelve or more months at hospital work. In order that these things *(Continued on Page 8)*

St. Vincent Hospital's newspaper in 1931 featured Harriett Osborn's graduation (Photo courtesy Providence Archives, Seattle)

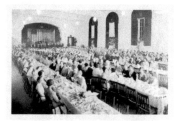

St. Vincent Nurses Alumnae banquet 1930. Annual banquets occurred every year for more than 100 years.

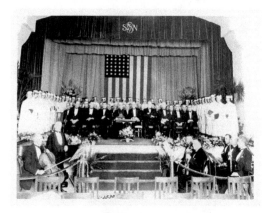

St. Vincent School of Nursing graduation, 1931

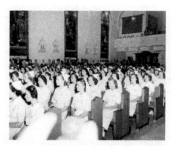

Capping ceremony, circa 1950 ©Oregonian Publishing Co. All rights reserved. Reprinted with permission.

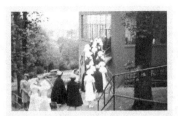

*Filing into the Capping Ceremony, circa 1950 ©Oregonian
Publishing Co. All rights reserved. Reprinted with permission.*

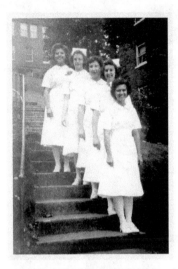

Dee Rennie Wallo (in front) lines up with classmates in 1945

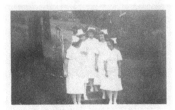

Dee and friends gather in front of the Nurses' Home in 1943

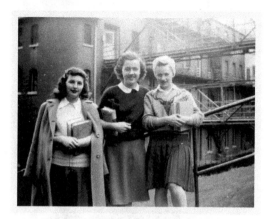

Inarose Zuelke (center) with classmates, circa 1947 (used with permission from the Zuelke Family).

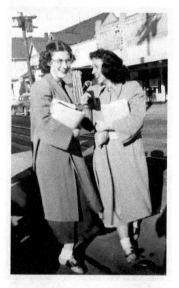

Roommates Joan Dove (left) and Dorothy Vardanega, 1952 (used with permission from the Raglione Family)

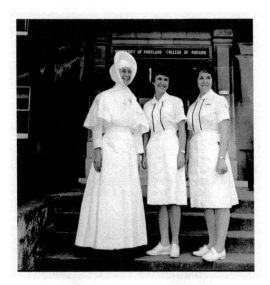

Sr. Bayless and students, circa 1950s (Photo courtesy Providence Archives, Seattle)

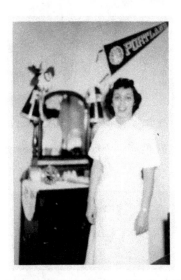

Dorothy Vardanega shows off her room in the Nurses' Home, circa 1948

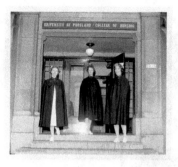

Showing off the capes in front of the Nurses' Home (Photo courtesy Providence Archives, Seattle)

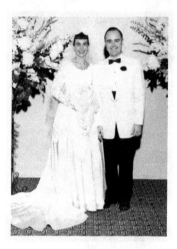

Ann and Jim Blickle's wedding day (used with permission from the Blickle family)

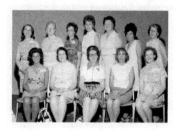

Dee's classmates on their 30th anniversary

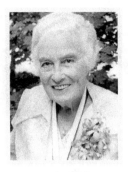

Harriett Osborn Jeckell, 1977

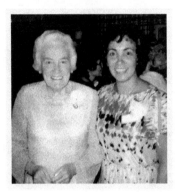

Ozzy and Dorothy Kennedy at Homecoming, circa late 1970s

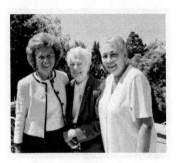

(From left) Dee, Sr. Rita and Dorothy Kennedy getting ready for Homecoming, 2010

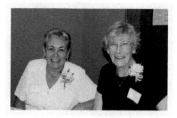

Dorothy Kennedy and Joan Raglione at Homecoming, circa 2005

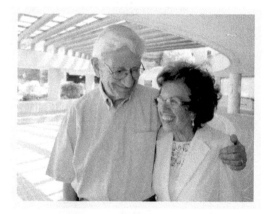

Dr. Ugo Raglione and Dee celebrate Homecoming, circa 2012

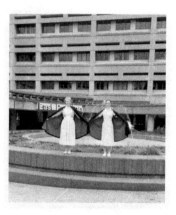

Delanie Strauss and Allie Potter, model old uniforms at Homecoming (photo in front of East Pavilion at St. Vincent)

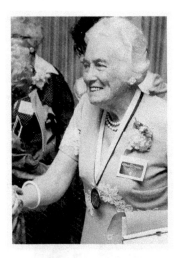

Harriett Osborn Jeckell is honored with a medal at Homecoming
1977

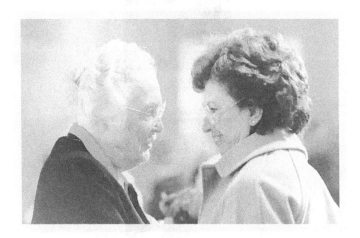

Harriett Osborn Jeckell and Dee Wallo share a laugh, 1990

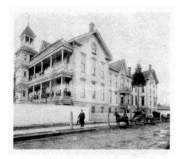

The first St. Vincent Hospital in Northwest Portland opened in 1875 (Photo courtesy Providence Archives, Seattle)

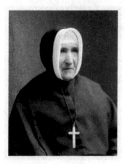

Mother Joseph (Photo courtesy Providence Archives, Seattle)

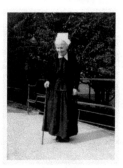

Rose Philpot was the first graduate in 1893 of the St. Vincent Training School

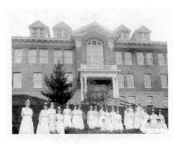

St. Vincent Training School, Class of 1909

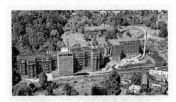

*An aerial view of the second St. Vincent Hospital, located in
Portland's west hills, circa 1960s (Photo courtesy Providence
Archives, Seattle)*

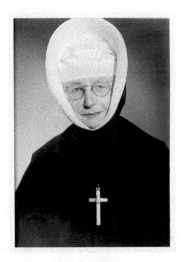

*Sister Genevieve de Nanterre, RN (Born Marie Verena
Gauthier), 1950 (Photo courtesy Providence Archives, Seattle)*

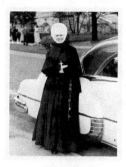

Sr. Mary Laureen poses for a photo, circa 1960s (Photo courtesy of the Raglione Family)

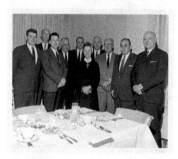

Sr. Mary Laureen poses with the all-male St. Vincent Medical Foundation, late 1960s (Photo courtesy Providence Archives, Seattle)

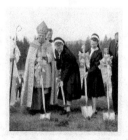

Archbishop Howard blesses the land prior to groundbreaking for the third St. Vincent Hospital, 1968 (Photo courtesy Providence Archives, Seattle)

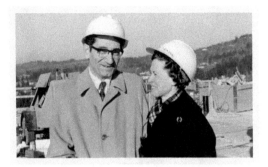

Dr. Ugo Raglione and Sister Mary Laureen discuss the building site of the third hospital (Photo courtesy Providence Archives, Seattle)

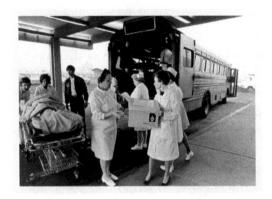

Moving day, January 31, 1971 (Photo courtesy Providence Archives, Seattle)

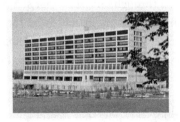

A postcard depicts the new hospital shortly after it opens in 1971 (Photo courtesy Providence Archives, Seattle)

THE NOTORIOUS 2 NORTH

Dee looked around with a sigh as she thought 2 North was just the same as she left it. Though it was evolving into more of a men's surgical ward, it held the promise of lots of work, including heavy patients to lift and help recover. There was never enough time to get everything done. Nevertheless, she went back to work, humming to herself, happy to be skipping down familiar halls again alongside the nuns. Dee's short legs moved as fast as they could down the hallway, her hat perched on her thick black curls. As the head nurse now at the age of 25, she watched as the nursing students shuttled through. She did what she could to mentor them, and connected with many. Even though they were younger than she was, they had the shared bond of St. Vincent Nursing School that automatically fused their lives together.

It was 1949, and Dee realized she was pregnant. She continued working, keeping her secret close—nurses were not allowed to work at the hospital while pregnant and she was wondering how she was going to support them, with Ed going to school full-time, eager to get his degree. Dee figured she was on limited time and could work until she really started showing.

The plan didn't quite go the way Dee had thought. One day while working, she paused, put a hand on her abdomen and told a coworker she was going upstairs. She didn't return. Dee entered the obstetrics department and gave birth at seven months to the couple's first child, a boy. Though he was tiny, he lived, but spent his first month in an incubator. His arrival was so early, most people were shocked and hadn't even guessed Dee was pregnant. Since even Dee and Ed were caught unaware of the baby's imminent arrival, they hadn't chosen a name yet. Dee's mother, ever-practical, suggested they name their son after both of them.

December 27 was a big day—the couple were planning to bring Edward Dee home. It was also their wedding anniversary. And lastly, Ed was sworn in by Chief James Fleming at the Portland Police Bureau. Thinking it was a short-term solution to their funding problems, Ed had decided to become a police officer because he would earn a paycheck immediately, even while being trained. He began working nights while finishing school at the University of Portland. After getting his degree, however, he realized he relished helping people and he was good at his job. He thought he would stay awhile working as a police officer. He stayed 35 years.

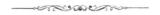

IT WAS NOW THE EARLY 1950S, AND DEE FELT FORTUNATE to have two great student nurses assigned to her who she really enjoyed: Dorothy Vardanega and Joan Dove. Dorothy and Dee soon bonded quickly. Dorothy had grown up in Portland, too, and looked like she could be sisters with Dee. Petite with black hair and olive skin, she loved to laugh and was gregarious. Dorothy's roommate at the school, Joan Dove, was also from Southeast Portland. Joan was quieter than Dorothy, but still rounded out the trio with her quick wit. Dorothy secretly told Dee that Joan was brilliant—she barely had to crack a book, reported Dorothy, who said she herself needed to be up all night studying just to keep up. Dee shook her head, silently empathetic, as she also had to study hard. Joan seemingly sailed through every test, getting the highest grades with ease.

Soon, the three noticed a new intern who seemed to be a fixture around 2 North, even if he didn't have a patient. A Portland native, Ugo Raglione was also born of Italian immigrants. Tall and lanky, he had black hair and big black glasses. He perched on the stool at the chart desk, often taking longer than normal to peruse the charts. Wondering which student nurse he was interested in, Dorothy or Joan, Dee simply shrugged and made use of him, having him sign orders and whatever else she needed. Methodical, "Rags," as he became known, talked slowly, choosing his words carefully. He had a big wide grin and an even bigger sense of humor, albeit a very dry one. He would draw out a story with plenty of detail and witty observations. Dee loved having Rags around, and she watched in fascination until she figured out the subject of his interest.

RAGS AND JOAN WERE MARRIED IN 1953, JUST A YEAR AFTER she graduated.

Meanwhile, Dorothy also graduated and joined Dee on 2 North, working alongside her now as great friends. There were 50 beds in total now: a few single rooms, some double rooms, and many four- and six-bed wards. There were just the two nurses assigned to 2 North, with two aides and an orderly.

As the head nurse, Dee would politely ask Dorothy at the start of each shift, "Which side do you want?"

Dorothy recalled later that she really wanted to respond, "What the hell does it matter?" Instead, Dorothy would simply shrug and take a side, digging in and working hard. She knew her day would be filled with running, lifting, and caring for some 25 patients with minimal help. She would watch Dee sail by doing the same thing; neither complained.

A third nurse, Ann Clark, supplemented the two, working on days that Dorothy or Dee had off. Ann had been a St. Vincent cadet, wearing her hat with its black stripe proudly. A short, stout woman with cat-eye glasses perched on her round face and a head of brown curls, she had a quick wit and a sharp tongue.

Ann loved to laugh and was known for her antics. Barreling down the hall and into the patients' rooms, she was a workhorse, and Dee was thankful to have her. One day, Dee was trying to lift a heavy man to get him back into the right position in bed to ease pressure on his wounded leg. The man, unconscious, was oblivious to Dee's struggle. Frustrated, Dee called Ann, who came quickly to her aid, grabbing and pulling. Suddenly, Dee began laughing so hard she let go of the patient, doubling over, clutching her stomach. Ann kept pulling, her hat askew and her face red.

Breathless, she indignantly finally asked, "What are you laughing about?"

Dee, trying to talk, finally gasped, "You're pulling on my leg, not the patient's."

Ann, never one to let anyone or anything rattle her, raised one eyebrow and retorted, "Well, I was wondering why he was wearing hose!"

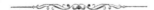

As time progressed, the 2 North crew became renowned for their thorough care. Nurses were added and word spread quickly that the staff who worked 2 North were impeccable, in part because Dee was exacting and expected them to work hard—but only as hard as she did. It also became known as the place to have fun, despite the heavy workload.

The 2 North unit also became legendary for the antics of the close-knit zany group. One such member was Mary Schmidt, the unit secretary. Known as Schmidty to friends, she was a tall blonde who loved to laugh and had a penchant for boots and short skirts, showing off her shapely legs. Big-hearted Schmidty would take care of anything for anyone and kept the place humming efficiently.

The patients of 2 North sometimes were men who were recovering from surgeries. For others, the unit was merely a brief detox stopover on the way to the county jail. Dee routinely called the jail for a pickup, and two police officers would soon show up and cart their man away. More than once, a patient/prisoner would simply jump from the second-story window to the bushes below to scramble down the driveway to freedom. The 2 North "medicine cabinet" grew, now full of alcohol bottles taken off the patients. When the cupboard couldn't close, it was time to throw a party at someone's house—BYOB took on a vastly different meaning.

The hospital was busier than ever and continued to grow. A modern cafeteria was added in the early 1950s. A subsequent fund-raising campaign was successful, with even the hospital employees contributing $20,000. It enabled the hospital to build an east wing in 1957, bringing patient capacity to 421 beds. The expansion included a modern emergency and physical therapy departments, a new nursery (including exam rooms and isolation nursery for premature babies), a new recovery room, a 42-bed pediatrics department, a wing with 17 additional beds for maternity, and admitting and business offices. The project cost $1.25 million, and the hospital was transformed. The nursing school continued, but now there was also a school for nurse anesthesiologists, lab technicians and x-ray technicians.

The hospital also added many new doctors, most of them returning from the war. One of the nurses' favorite doctors was Dr. Ambrose Shields. Dr. Shields, known as Bucky to everyone for some unknown reason, was a short, stout Irishman, with a head of dark wavy hair, parted in the middle. He hailed from Kansas and ventured west with his wife, Alice, after hearing from family that Oregon was a nice place and St. Vincent was a good place to work. He had worked closely with Dr. Joyce from Dee's training days, but then had to ship out to serve as a medic in the war.

Returning to Oregon, Bucky resumed his practice and was a mainstay at St. Vincent Hospital. He had a fatherly fondness for the nurses, and would often sit in the charting area, sharing information about new techniques he was learning and recalling his days during the war when they had little medicine and advancements to help the wounded. Although Dr. Shields had seen his share of atrocities during the war, he liked to tell a story about when he met General Patton.

Dee and her friends crowded around as he talked about serving at a hospital in Sicily. There had been a recent bombing nearby, injuring many soldiers. Soon after, General Patton arrived for a special ceremony 'to pin on Purple Hearts. Dr. Shields directed him to one of his patients and watched with awe when the general kneeled down beside the young man and pinned on the Purple Heart. When saluting the young man, tears streamed down Patton's face. He then whispered quietly to each critically burned sailor, who were wrapped up like mummies in an attempt to heal their burns.

Before leaving that day, General Patton took Dr. Shields aside, asking if he had any whiskey. Dr. Shields told him regrettably they only had odds and ends of alcohol—some Marsala wine, a little eggnog and brandy mix. Patton just shook his head. The next day, three cases of whiskey arrived, compliments of the General.

DR. SHIELDS WAS JUST ONE OF AN INFLUX OF DOCTORS coming to St. Vincent Hospital from all over the country, drawn by the hospital's excellent reputation. Medicine was moving at lightning speed, and what Dee didn't realize was that 2 North was about to become a specialized all-in-one recovery room and intensive care unit.

About this time, a young Japanese-American doctor arrived on the scene. Dr. Toshio Inahara, later known simply as "Toke" to only those in his inner circle, hailed from Tacoma, Washington. Eventually his family traveled to Oregon, where he graduated from the University of Oregon Medical School. At the onset of World War II, he and his family were uprooted and forced to re-establish themselves in Eastern Oregon. When the war ended, Dr. Inahara finished his residency at St. Vincent, and then completed a two-year fellowship in vascular surgery at Massachusetts General Hospital before returning to Portland to work.

Dr. Inahara began performing vascular surgeries that no one had seen before at St. Vincent. In his 2005 book, *A Nisei, Right Place, Right Time*, Dr. Inahara discussed how the specialty was in its infancy in the 1950s, with surgeries only performed at major hospitals. He knew it was time for St. Vincent to take on these progressive vascular surgery techniques and if his patients survived, he needed educated nurses to assist in their recovery. Remarkably, only a few nurses had ever been trained to take blood pressures.

Dr. Inahara quietly took Dee aside to inform her that his patients would recover in 2 North. Wide-eyed, she respectfully tried to explain she did not know the first thing about taking care of vascular patients. Firm in his resolve that she could do it, he patiently taught her how to take femoral and posterior tibial pulses, and other important skills. He was exacting, difficult and the best teacher she could ever ask for. She eagerly took her new knowledge and taught others.

Advances in cardiac surgery were also coming to St. Vincent. Dr. Albert Starr, an innovative cardiovascular surgeon, had been making headlines at the open-heart surgery program at the University of Oregon Medical School. Dr. Starr had performed the first pediatric open-heart surgery at the University Hospital, and collaborated with M. Lowell Edwards on an artificial valve that could replace diseased heart valves. The Starr-Edwards valve was an amazing breakthrough in cardiac medicine, resulting in thousands of patients to seek surgery in Oregon. Dr. Starr, Dr. James Wood and their colleagues were knee-deep in cardiac patients.

The surgeons expanded and brought the first open-heart surgery program to St. Vincent Hospital. Dee suddenly found herself at the forefront of this revolutionary time in cardiac surgical history and was able to witness the first surgery and care for the patient. Unfortunately, the patient did not make it, but Dee suddenly became the de facto new cardiac recovery head nurse.

The surgeons began performing two to three cardiac surgeries a week, and additional surgeons arrived to learn from the masters.

Dee was enthralled with cardiac surgery. Maybe it was her own heart issues or possibly it was the thrill of being in on this groundbreaking medicine, Dee anxiously learned all she could.

Years later, the hospital became the first private hospital to feature a coronary intensive care unit. In the meantime, Room 232 was turned into open heart intensive care with Dee and her nurses taking care of the patients.

During this new influx of cardiac patients, a problem emerged with one doctor involved. This doctor in question had a foul mouth, and he would be the first to acknowledge it. Maybe it was the pressure of lives on the line or the national attention the program was now receiving, but he felt the need to dress-down nurses rudely he perceived were not doing their jobs correctly.

Dee wasn't going to have it, not in her ward. She had been accommodating, taking the high-risk, high-maintenance patients and her nurses were doing the best they could. No one, but *no one,* was going to correct them except her, and she made that pretty clear to the doctors. Apparently, this new doctor had not received that message yet.

Dee did what a skilled manager should do—she took care of it with the finality of a door slamming. Dragging the doctor into the linen closet to preserve his ego, she grabbed hold of his arm. "Listen here," she said with her famous opening. "You will not speak that way to my nurses or use that language around here."

No one knows to this day what else was said. The doctor and Dee emerged from the closet with him nodding toward her. "Mrs. Wallo," he said. "Doctor," she nodded back, pivoting toward the chart desk where the staff suddenly busied themselves with charts, trying their hardest not to smirk, except for Schmidty, who laughed as she typed.

Later, Dee discovered that another young doctor had a bit of an impulse anger issue. This doctor could be charming and witty as he laughed and told jokes. Other times, if he became angry, he would take it out on the nurses, throwing charts at them—even if they were uninvolved. The nurses learned how to duck and dodge the incoming metal charts lobbed through the air toward them. When Dee learned of this, she quickly dispatched herself to take care of the situation.

Into the linen closet they went, now her unofficial office.

"Listen here," she said, grabbing the doctor by the elbow, leaning into his surprised face. "You throw one more chart and you are out of here, understand?" This time she just narrowed her eyes at him, gave him one last long look and walked out. The doctor stood there for some time before gathering himself together, closing the door quietly and walking away. No chart was ever thrown again, and the doctor quietly held his temper in check.

The staff said later that no one stuck up for them as much as Dee, especially when it came to doctors who hadn't yet realized that most times, the experienced nurses knew more about nursing care and recovery than they ever could.

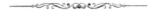

THE CARDIAC DOCTOR AND THE CHART-THROWING DOCTOR weren't the only ones to receive Dee's wrath. Jim Blickle was a doctor of internal medicine, who had married Ann Smith, the hilarious nursing student from the famous bedpan flusher incident. Short and stout, with a receding hairline, Dr. Blickle was a popular doctor who cared deeply for his patients. He often performed house calls, never able to refuse anyone's request and always keeping his patient's care at the forefront. The problem was his lack of performing the necessary duties associated with the paperwork involved. Dee often chased him down to remind him he had not updated his charts or orders.

Dee had another issue with Dr. Blickle that centered on

his apparent inability to say no. He had a kind heart and responded to those who needed him during his time off, even on holidays. Frequently, Dee wished he was not so generous in spirit, especially regarding one specific patient who often was hospitalized because of a stomach ulcer. This patient was just plain mean. He was condescending to the nurses, fighting with them, and was generally a "pill to take care of," according to Dee. One day, Dee took Dr. Blickle aside. "Listen here," she started in, "Never admit that man again into my ward. We are done being abused by this patient."

Soon after, Dee was doing rounds and glanced into a room. There was Dr. Blickle, bent over a patient. She looked more closely, narrowing her eyes suspiciously, trying to see what was going on. As Dr. Blickle moved, the patient came into her view and sure enough—it was the banned abuser. As Dr. Blickle emerged from the room and saw Dee, his eyes widened behind his black glasses. Dr. Blickle did what anyone would do in his position: he ran.

Dee ran after him, her short legs trying to keep up with his. Down the corridor they went, round the bend where Dee almost knocked one nun over, flying past her. "Sorry, Sister," she panted, waving, but not breaking stride. Dr. Blickle ran to the perfect safety net: the Doctor's Lounge. Not even Dee would enter that sacred ground. She stood outside the door that had swung shut, eyeing the placard with a frown. After a few minutes, she walked away, her eyes still narrowed, her brow furrowed. She would catch up with him—it was only a matter of time.

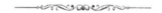

WHILE DEE WAS RUNNING, LIFTING, ORDERING AND managing the growth of her unit, she was just as busy at home.

Eight years after their son Edward's arrival, another son, Steve, was born in 1957. Steve was also a bit premature, but this time Dee disclosed her pregnancy and took time off. Dee, now 33 years old, enjoyed her two boys, getting down on the floor to play with them, feeling so fortunate to have them. However, the family still financially needed her paycheck and she loved her job. An older woman in the neighborhood who had cared for Edward offered to babysit Steve while she went back to work.

Not long after, Dee found herself pregnant with her third child, and discovered to her ire she could not keep it a secret. Ed's partner at work, also named Ed, had a wife who was pregnant too and due remarkably at the same time as Dee. The local newspaper found out about these two officers who had walked the beat together for five years and the coincidence with their wives' pregnancies. They ran the story with a promise of a Grand Prize (diapers, formula, etc.) to whoever delivered first. Dee's doctor had other ideas and after examining her, he made an appointment for her to come in for an induction. The night before Dee's appointment, the partner's wife called to say she was on her way to the hospital after the popular show *Playhouse 90* was over. She ultimately delivered first, winning the prize. To add insult to injury, while reading the newspaper the day after giving birth, Dee found out her new daughter had already been named. Apparently, when the reporter asked Ed the name of his new baby daughter, Ed panicked and thought of a name he had recently seen and liked: MaryJo. Never mind that Dee had wanted to name her baby Theresa or Terri after her mother if it was a girl. Dee could never get truly angry at her husband and instead, just shook her head and uttered what she usually said at times like this: "Oh, Ed."

Fortunately, another daughter came around three years later and Dee was able to have her Terri. This time when she had to leave the hospital during her pregnancy, Dr. Inahara provided an alternative. He employed her as a medical transcriptionist—a task Dee found tedious, carefully and laboriously checking a medical dictionary frequently. She was grateful to her old friend, but was eager to get back to patient care. She silently typed away in an office all day by herself, so lonely she once invited the postal worker to come in and sit down to talk with her.

For a woman who was never supposed to have children because of her damaged heart, Dee stubbornly refused that guidance, giving birth to Terri at the age of 38. "When is it going to stop?" sniffed her mother, Theresa.

The family had an idyllic life, their home in northeast Portland conveniently near Fernhill Park, the center of neighborhood activity. Dee's parents lived just two blocks to the east, and her Aunt Lena and Uncle Tony lived two blocks west. Both couples were a big help to the young family, especially with Dee working the 6:30 a.m. to 3:30 p.m. shift at 2 North, driving across town each day. Ed continued to work nights and Dee found herself a single mother during those years—trying her best to keep her children entertained with creative, inexpensive activities.

Unfortunately, she had given birth to four accident-prone kids. The family's big car was often seen pulling up to the hospital's emergency room for treatment of broken bones, cuts and other minor injuries. A window would soon fly open and one sister or another would poke her head out and shout: "Which one is it this time, Dee?"

One time Dee's drive to the ER wasn't so minor, however. Just a few days after New Year's, Ed and Dee's youngest child, Terri, who was just seven at the time, was playing. Teasing her brother, she grabbed his wallet, wanting him to chase her. She climbed onto her bunk bed and then jumped to the dresser. Terri's planned dive off the dresser—a maneuver she had landed successfully several times—did not go so well this time. Her arm was crushed behind her and she screamed for her parents. Running in, Ed took one look at her and knew it was bad. A seasoned first responder, he tore a nearby box in half, slid it under the arm and cradled their daughter. Dee drove to the hospital across town as fast as she could, with Ed holding Terri the whole way. This time Dee was frightened.

Steve and MaryJo bounced around in the back seat, excited about this unexpected car drive and unaware how upset their parents were. MaryJo, who now considered herself an expert after a minor break in her wrist the previous year, surmised out loud what would be done to her little sister. This made Terri suddenly begin to shriek.

The emergency room staff sprang into action, taking the child immediately for x-rays and then to an operating room. Ed was forced to take the other kids home, and Dee sat alone in the emergency room on the other side of healthcare and tried to be brave.

Doctors began pouring through the door—responding to the call that Dee Wallo's daughter had a serious injury. Dee was overwhelmed watching so many doctors and friends run through the door on a Saturday night. One doctor (ironically the one Dee had taken to the linen closet to discuss his foul mouth), came to sit with her now as a friend, trying to be reassuring as she signed authorization papers for the surgeons to amputate her child's arm if needed. The surgeons had been trying frantically to get a pulse in Terri's left arm and had been unsuccessful. "I'll go in if I need to," said the doctor sitting with Dee, "but Toke is a better vascular doctor," he admitted with modesty. As if on cue, as he was referenced, Dr. Inahara ran in, throwing aside his jacket. "How long has she been down?" he yelled, flying through the doors toward the OR.

Between Dr. Inahara's vascular skills and Dr. Tom Fagan's

orthopedic proficiencies, Terri's arm was saved. She recovered in the pediatric wing of the hospital for several weeks, enjoying the attention that being Dee Wallo's daughter brought. She recovered completely, a wicked scar being the only physical reminder of the accident. Dee, on the other hand, would remember that night for a long time.

Life went on with Dee working hard every day at the hospital and then coming home to her young family—a second job of sorts—but one that she loved. The kids knew her white Chevy—a successor to the midnight blue one—would roll up exactly at 4 p.m. each day and they couldn't wait to see that big smile.

Dee never let her work life intrude too invasively, except for the hour she needed occasionally to lie on the floor, her legs up against the wall, trying desperately to ease the ache. She would use that time to call Ann Clark and brief her on the patients—they went through them one by one, bed by bed, discussing ailments, prognosis and care. That done, she'd roll up, stand up slowly and begin her tasks at home.

Whether it was the demands at work or at home, Dee's heart issues finally made themselves apparent. She was diagnosed with heart failure, and for the first time saw a cardiologist and took medicine to manage it. It slowed her down temporarily, but soon she was back up and running and no one was the wiser. Dee remained head nurse at 2 North, working just as hard as she always did.

CHANGING TIMES—SISTER MARY
LAUREEN MAKES A MOVE

As medicine advanced, so did academics required for nurses, which meant the St. Vincent School of Nursing was changing. Though these brave, resilient and hardworking women had faced insurmountable challenges and kept the hospital running through the Depression, wars, pandemics, widespread influenza and disease, times were changing. Dee had watched the school change over the years, but it remained a constant source for graduating the best nurses.

In fact, back in 1949, the school had reached a professional milestone by becoming one of the first collegiate schools of nursing in the United States to receive full accreditation from the League of Nursing Education. The League singled out the school's state-of-the-art laboratory as one item that moved this decision.

In 1950, the League of Nursing had pressed gently for stronger academics. However, the University of Portland took a different direction, marketing courses in "charm" for its nursing students. In 1954, the local newspaper reported on this, showing photos of nursing students practicing their charm exercises, including poise, while also keeping up with their medical studies. These glamour classes instructed the girls on grooming, diction and what to do with their hands when they weren't working, rubbing backs or carrying bedpans.

One can only imagine the eye rolling Ozzy must have done over this marketing campaign, though it was an attempt to attract nursing students because of a nursing shortage. Ozzy told the local newspaper that nursing students and graduates were getting married quickly now that the war was over and wanting to raise children, leaving the profession behind. Once the students were enrolled, Ozzy took over and continued her role, now serving as the nursing arts instructor and nursing services director. However, things were changing in her personal life as well.

In 1958, Ozzy made the tough decision to retire to care selflessly for her ailing mother. Unfortunately, retirement meant a financial struggle for her as she was too young to qualify for Social Security and she had no pension from the hospital (a retirement fund was started in the 1960s). Eventually, upon the death of an aunt and uncle, Ozzy inherited a house on the Sandy River, just east of Portland. She loved the property, for it reminded her of her beloved Klondike with its roaring rivers and tall trees.

Ozzy rose every day, grateful for her humble life, and made her bed with the tight hospital corners she had so demanded from her nursing students. In her free time, she played the piano, ice-skated, and rode her bike to keep physically fit. She continued even after retirement to guide and form policies that focused on high standards. Ozzy served as president, vice president, board member and chair of every committee of the Oregon Nurses Association, and was on the board and committees of the Oregon League of Nursing. She served on the State Board of Nurse Licensure, community health planning committees, and on the board of the American Red Cross. However, with her departure from the school, there would be no more Ozzy's Girls.

Even more concerning, around the same time as Ozzy's departure, the League of Nursing issued a formal warning that if the St. Vincent Nursing School was to keep its accreditation, it must become an integral part of the University of Portland. To accomplish this, the school was forced to move physically to the University of Portland campus.

By 1963, the St. Vincent School of Nursing was shuttered and completely absorbed by the university. From 1894 to 1962, the St. Vincent School of Nursing or the University of Portland College of Nursing at St. Vincent graduated more than 1,600 students, but the unique era was over.

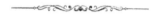

DEE, STILL THE HEAD NURSE OF 2 NORTH, SWALLOWED THIS new development with resignation. While she was thrilled to see advancements in medicine and couldn't wait to learn more, there was one trait Dee readily admitted she could not shake: She was resistant to change. Like most people, she found change daunting and she loved her routine, the rhythm of her hospital and her cherished coworkers. Over the next decade, Dee was to find this was slowly going to evolve and she hung on with the tenacity she was known for.

In the 1960s, the Sisters of Providence still retained control. A string of sisters, from Mother Petronilla to Mother Flora Mary—with others in between—continued to oversee the flourishing hospital.

The director of nursing services was now Sister Mary Laureen. Growing up as Rita Ferschweiler on a farm in rural Oregon with five siblings, young Rita devoted herself to serving others; she joined the Sisters of Providence, taking the name Mary Laureen. She earned a bachelor's degree and later a Master in Nursing Service and Administration, and worked in a few other Providence hospitals on the West Coast before returning to Oregon. She started as a surgical nurse, quickly climbing the ranks.

Whether she was channeling Mother Joseph or Mother Mary Theresa, or simply drawing from her own inspiration, Sister Mary Laureen was a take-action kind of nun. She and Dee saw eye-to-eye on that score.

"She was a great boss," Dee once said. "Very supportive, a good listener, and always laughing. She had a great sense of humor. I can't stress enough her warmth and interest in everyone."

Meanwhile, the hospital was the busiest it had ever been. In 1962 alone, the hospital cared for 25,000-plus patients. That same year, the Council on Medical Education and Hospitals of the American Medical Association approved St. Vincent's program for four-year residencies in pathology and surgery, three-year residencies in medicine, two-year residencies in general practice, and one-year internships. St. Vincent had the distinction of being the only private hospital in Oregon to be approved for the four-year surgery and two-year general practice programs. It was an exciting time for those working at St. Vincent Hospital, while also maintaining a family environment. Employees participated in regular off-duty social events, such as dances and picnics, and everyone knew everyone else's business like a small-town.

Life was about to change for Sister Mary Laureen, though. One day in 1964, a letter was delivered from the Sisters of Providence Mother House, still in Montreal, promptly naming her administrator. When it was delivered, Sister Mary Laureen was found praying in the chapel. She ran downstairs and said, "There must be some mistake." She soon learned it was not an error, and now Sister Mary Laureen would become the youngest administrator to be given this responsibility in the Sisters of Providence network.

Whether it was her personality, her open-door policy (to anyone from the janitor to nurses and doctors), Sister Mary Laureen hit the ground running. The staff enjoyed telling stories about her—including her secret habit of slipping out to pitch baseballs on the rough patch of land that had served as a baseball diamond behind the hospital when she was stressed—an activity that brought her comfort, reminding her of days on the farm with her many siblings. Sister Mary Laureen was often found in her office at midnight hand-writing commendation notes to hospital personnel, and was known to get up at odd hours, such as 2 a.m., just to have coffee with the night staff so they could provide feedback. Sister Mary Laureen also frequently responded in person to the latest facility crisis, such as a sewer break at the aging hospital, no matter what time it was.

She soon sought advice during weekly coffees with some of the doctors. Maybe it was the continual crises, but Sister Mary Laureen felt more change was needed. She once wrote about this time and explosion of scientific knowledge that was driving business to the hospital:

"Once upon a time, there was a hospital on the hill in northwest Portland. We had a beautiful view of the city; we had an excellent medical and nursing staff; we had good patient care. But we had run out of room. Technology was just beginning to push the 'what is' for the 'what ought to be' for 'what had to be' if St. Vincent was to continue as a premier hospital. We didn't say 'health care facility' then. We were a hospital and didn't even want the title medical center. We wanted to be known as a hospital; that was our history, our reputation. And like the Lord, we looked at what we had, and it was good."

Indeed, the hospital was becoming increasingly taxed. Despite the renovations made in the 1950s, the hospital had simply outgrown itself and was bursting at the seams. The surgery suite had been refurbished to care for the growing number of cardiac patients. The intensive care unit was assembled on the fourth floor—once called the catacombs. And the hospital's beautiful chapel on the sixth floor had been converted for medical records, while the chapel had moved to a former dining room for the sisters on the seventh floor. Meanwhile, the issue surrounding parking had reached a crisis. Parking was minimal at the hospital, and employees and visitors had to arrive early or face the long walk up the hill. In addition, the northwest area of Portland had become increasingly popular and now featured shops and restaurants, which made parking even down the hill challenging.

"There were so many things we needed to do," Sister Mary Laureen said at the time in an interview with the *Oregon Journal*. "Some rooms had no water. We already had reduced the number of beds to make space for new equipment and expanded departments. Open heart surgery was coming into the picture and we had no room for it."

It was time for drastic measures, and Sister Mary Laureen wasn't the only one who knew it. To help plan for the future, she started what was later called simply, "The 7 a.m. Committee."

Dr. Ugo Raglione was a regular at these informal brainstorming sessions. Rags and Joan had left Portland while he served in the Navy as the chief of surgery for a naval base at Mare Island, California. Now they were back with a burgeoning family, and he was a surgeon at St. Vincent.

The group talked about where to build, how big to build it, and what the needs were.

"Sister Mary Laureen was a good listener," Dr. Raglione once remarked. "She was willing to listen to new ideas, and she insisted others listen, too. "In fact, she wouldn't close her door—even when there was work to be done," Rags added with a slight eye roll.

Dr. Raglione's partner in his practice, Dr. Arch Diack, was also a member of the 7 a.m. Committee. He and his brother, Sam, were renowned physicians in Portland. Arch had served in WWII, as a physician in North Africa and France. He returned to Portland after the war, and found his way to St. Vincent, serving as chief of staff for a time. Dr. Diack had asked Rags to join his practice when Rags finished his residency.

Like Rags, Dr. Diack was a good person for the committee. Innovative and forward-thinking, he would later be known for being the first person to conceive of an automated electronic defibrillator. With his partner, Dr. W. Stanley Welborn, Dr. Diack developed the portable Cardiac Automatic Resuscitative Device (CARD) that could diagnose a heart that was stopped or fibrillating, and deliver an electrical shock capable of restarting it. Known as the "Heart-Aid," it was programmed to diagnose specific problems and designed for temporary use by laypeople in emergency situations before professional care could be administered. This kind of innovative thinking was needed to re-envision the hospital's future.

The 7 a.m. Committee did a lot of coffee drinking, a lot of arguing and a whole lot of dreaming. Sister Mary Laureen, with her calm manner, quietly steered the helm.

All that listening eventually led Sister Mary Laureen to realize it was now time to think about paying for the construction of this dream. She started a lay advisory board, which formally became the St. Vincent Hospital Foundation in 1969.

Finding a new home was complex—few people on the 7 a.m. Committee agreed on the location. Some doctors stubbornly insisted it should be downtown, while others looked west of the old hospital.

Sister Mary Laureen talked about those days in a paper she wrote about the project:

> "I recall visiting a site that overlooked Mt. Calvary Cemetery, a very nice piece of property. One of those sisters, who is now listening from Heaven, was horrified that we would even consider a site where patients could see a cemetery. I told her that maybe we could make a deal with the cemetery and save some money for families. That was not funny [to the sister], and she insisted that more people be included to make the decision in choosing a proper place to move."

Sister Mary Laureen kept looking, and the group finally agreed on the purchase of 40 acres of land on Southwest Barnes Road. Technically a Portland address, the new hospital would be in Washington County—just a couple miles from neighboring Multnomah County—where the current hospital resided. Traveling up the hill from the current hospital on a one-lane road shaded by giant evergreens, and yes, through Mt. Calvary Cemetery, this new area was largely undeveloped and unpopulated. This part of Washington County had just a smattering of small neighborhoods with newer homes. Highway 217, now an extremely busy roadway, was just a couple of lanes with stoplights.

People lined up outside that proverbially open door to tell Sister there would be too many traffic problems, the site wasn't right, and the plans needed adjusting. Sister Mary

Laureen stubbornly held her ground, reminiscent of Mother Mary Theresa's desire to move the hospital west and the pushback she received.

On a bright Sunday morning, March 31, 1968, a ground-breaking ceremony featured Sister Mary Laureen surrounded by a sea of men. Not forgetting their Catholic roots, Archbishop Robert J. Dwyer was on hand to sprinkle holy water on the ground. "My main concern is not with the physical structure, but with the spirit that engendered the work," he said.

Sister Mary Laureen later wrote to employees:

> "The ceremonies were meaningful and inspiring and the beautiful spirit that pervaded the crowd was the same spirit that pervades St. Vincent every day—a spirit of love and concern without which we would be foolish to continue our building program. Bricks and mortar can form a building; it takes devoted and dedicated people to make a hospital."

Sister Mary Laureen was going to need a lot of those people she had referenced, for she and her group of volunteers had big dreams. A July 1, 1970, article in *The Oregonian* detailed the 10-year, $50 million development plan, which was announced by the St. Vincent Foundation at the Sheraton Motor Inn. Glenn L. Jackson, president of the foundation, made the announcement. With him was Oregon Governor Tom McCall and former United States Vice President Hubert H. Humphrey, who had flown in to address the meeting of 400 potential donors.

The plans were called an "imaginative concept." The ambitious plan not only outlined the specifics of a hospital, but many other needs, including two office buildings; a cancer unit; an education center; extended care pavilion; diagnostic and treatment services; mental health center; heart center and cardiovascular special procedures department; new housing, including minimal quarters for self-care patients, students of medicine and allied health professions, and transient patient relatives; pulmonary function; laboratory; burn center; and extensive parking.

As with any massive project, there were meetings and compromises, technical problems and more. Of course, there were funding issues as well. Sister Mary Laureen once said her cloudy crystal ball did not show all the challenges she would ultimately face, but she persevered. She credited Dr. Raglione as the driving force.

Sister Mary Laureen had learned a few things about Rags, and she soon realized he was the answer to her prayers. What many people didn't know was that Rags was also an engineer. After graduating from high school, Rags began working in the drafting room of Bingham-Willamette Iron & Steel. He continued working there through college, becoming an engineer prior to going to medical school. During medical school, he spent half a day at the plant and the other half in school or at the hospital. During the war, Rags served as a marine engineer specializing in mechanical systems on ships. He continued working as a consultant while also being a prominent surgeon.

Sister Mary Laureen seized on this opportunity that she felt dropped directly from heaven and promptly put Rags on staff to oversee the planning and design of the hospital with the simple title of "building coordinator."

Sister Mary Laureen noted later that Rags simply took charge and ran the show. He embraced the new project, deeply interested in developing the site. Rags essentially put his practice on hold for two years to accomplish the planning, design and construction project. It was a volunteer endeavor that was obviously near to his heart. Sister Mary Laureen appreciated his hard work and relied on his technical understanding of both design and construction and how to apply it to the hospital's medical needs.

Meanwhile, Rags had a new family home built right behind the hospital. Though he did not design it, it wasn't surprising that he made modifications to the plans. However, he focused more on the hospital, making sure he was available for every critical construction decision and sometimes even the not-so-crucial construction tasks at the new hospital. A perfectionist, he often showed up unannounced to watch workers complete a project, carefully inspecting their work. Mother Joseph and Rags were kindred spirits in that way.

Sister Mary Laureen leaned on Rags for one more favor: to be the liaison with other physicians, as well as staff members, who were still horrified about the idea of moving to what was considered the country.

In fact, Dee and some of the 2 North crew decided they would go see for themselves how far away the new hospital was. After work, the group had gone out to dinner and the idea was born to do a little exploring. Dee found her car filled with 2 North staff, including one of her nurses, Joan O'Keeffe Currie, who was a gregarious woman. Joan was talking and talking and her straight man, Schmidty, was making side comments and observations as the group sailed over the hill westbound. However, as they got near Mt. Calvary Cemetery, they suddenly encountered thick fog. Dee slowed the big car to a crawl, and they crept along silently on the still road. Dee couldn't see a thing and could tell by the silence in the car, especially from Joan, she was not the only one worried.

"Pull the car over, Mrs. Wallo," Schmidty said quietly.

Dee obediently did so without question.

Schmidty sprung out the car door. Wearing her bright-colored coat, she grabbed a scarf which she waved high into the air as she marched down the road. Dee, still at the wheel, inched the car behind Schmidty. The passengers sat holding their breaths. The parade continued slowly down Barnes Road until suddenly the fog lifted just as quickly as it had come. Schmidty jumped back into the car as laughter and shouts rang out. They only had a few yards left when they pulled up to what was fast becoming their new hospital. The group was once again silent as they stared at what appeared to be an enormous building. Dee turned the car around and they drove back home, this time with no parade or laughter, but daunted by the changes that were on their horizon.

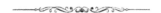

MOVING DAY FINALLY ARRIVED. IT WAS FOGGY AND overcast on Sunday, January 31, 1971. The planning for the move had started more than six months prior, with the moving company even asking for an office at the old hospital to better coordinate things. The hospital had intentionally reduced its patient population to prepare for the big day.

The hospital wasn't the only thing that was going to look different. Post Vatican II, Sister Mary Laureen had joined other nuns in shedding their habits. Dressed in a simple skirt and top, which was covered by a white lab coat, her brown curls were visible now with no head piece. She got into an ambulance with a few of the patients and bid farewell to the old hospital. When she emerged from the ambulance, she looked up to see the $20 million 400-bed, more than 500,000-square-foot, nine-story hospital, waiting for its first patients. Inside, Rags and his sons quickly hung crucifixes to patient rooms and inspected everything in one last round before the chaos hit.

Most of St. Vincent Hospital's entire staff of 400, half of them nurses, were on duty that day. One-third of them were at the new hospital, one-third were readying the 82 patients who were moved, and one-third tended to the traveling patients. The 40th Aeromedical Evacuation Squadron also helped employees and volunteers with the move.

The day went off smoothly thanks to the extensive planning. The oldest patient moved was Sister Johanna Sibernagel, 101, and the youngest one was Rebecca Nichols, who came in her incubator and was said to have slept the whole way. The move was completed in three-and-half hours, and despite the uprooting, the participants were jovial, dining on breakfast at the old hospital and lunch at the new.

Sister Mary Laureen walked the long hallways filled with green, gold and rust carpet. She watched as the modern elevators began dinging, as if they too were celebrating with a brief spurt of joy. She looked out over the courtyard and saw the hospital's bell, which had been carefully placed there. A gift from the Northwest missionary priest Reverend Louis Verhaag to the Sisters of Providence at the first St. Vincent Hospital, it was later moved to the hospital in the foothills, where its peals could be heard throughout Portland's West Side. Now it had been moved a third time, nestled into the outside nook near the hospital lobby. Its inscription is simple: 1884—St. Vincent, Pray for Us.

Sister Mary Laureen, who had spent almost seven years on the move project, smiled satisfactorily and said: "The spirit of the hospital is here now."

AND DEE? SHE WAS FOUND AT THE OLD HOSPITAL, TEARS IN her eyes, packing up last-minute records and walking the halls of 2 North, once called her domain. A patient, due to go home, perched on a stool and tried to cheer her.

She eventually drove up the hill, through Mt. Calvary Cemetery, where there was no fog that day. She looked to her right and saw a statue of the Virgin Mary, to whom she had often prayed. She saw that as a positive sign and drove on, her heart lighter.

Once Dee got to the new hospital, she wandered the halls in wonder. The carpet and paint smelled so new. She couldn't believe how massive the building was, and she laughed that every time there was a ding, someone at the chart desk would pick up the phone, not realizing it was the elevator. She went to the new chapel, essentially a conference room with some chairs, but already a sanctuary. She sat down and closed her eyes for a minute, trying to soak it all in.

Sister Mary Laureen later recalled that life simply continued as if nothing had occurred: "I remember that Dr. Zuelke delivered a baby [Angela Christine Heft] at the new St. Vincent that Sunday afternoon [move day] and one patient left us to go to heaven. So...life begins and ends, no matter what else is going on."

And yes, life continued. Even though the new modern hospital was well-equipped and well-planned thanks to Dr. Raglione, who was now chairman of general and vascular surgery, the old guard still missed their former building and special time they had all shared within its walls.

Dee's 2 North had been transformed to 7 East at the new hospital where she, now in her late 40s, continued her work as now the unit director—a title that made her roll her eyes. "I'm a head nurse no matter what they call me," she said out loud to whoever questioned her new nametag. She still worked alongside many of Ozzy's Girls—Joan O'Keeffe Currie, Dorothy Vardanega Kennedy, and many others. Schmidty was also still there to ensure the unit ran smoothly and with laughter.

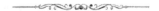

PARALLEL TO THE HOSPITAL'S MOVE, ED AND DEE DECIDED maybe it was time to move their household as well. "I'm not driving even farther to work," Dee said, eager to be able to spend as much time as possible with her growing children.

Ed agreed and incredibly bought their new home without Dee even seeing it. One day, he was driving past a house located behind the new St. Vincent. He anchored the car after being overwhelmed at the view of the western Cascades from the large windows in the open garage. He went to the front door, and in his usual fashion, talked himself into the house and had coffee with the aging couple who admitted they had been thinking about moving.

Dee simply shook her head when he told her. "Oh, Ed," she said, as she always did, ultimately laughing.

"You won't have to do anything," Ed assured her. "I'll get it all done." That promise was something he couldn't keep, however. Prior to moving, as he was cleaning out the garage attic, Ed fell off a ladder. His son Steve found him lying on the floor of the garage and called for an ambulance. With broken ribs, Ed was now a patient in the new hospital. As Dee leveled him with a look, he picked up the phone meekly. Soon a crew of his officers and coworkers arrived, complete with a paddy wagon. They swarmed in, grabbed the family's furniture and boxes and made dozens of trips across town. Though their heart was in the right place trying to help their lieutenant, they were not experienced movers. Furniture and boxes were casually placed everywhere, creating a chaotic scene at the new home.

And though she talked big about avoiding the longer commute, Dee had tears in her eyes when she left her beloved home that the couple had built on Northeast 38th Street. Her son Edward held her tight as she looked at her soon to be ex-house, which held so many of the family's memories. When she arrived at her new home, she took one look at the mess and sank down on a box for just a minute to cry. The kids, meanwhile, ran outside to jump up and down on the deck, waving at their dad. Ed saw them and waved back from his bed on Dee's 7 East.

The family settled into their new home in the shadow of St. Vincent, where Dee walked to work in the snow if the roads were treacherous. The house was just a block away from Dr. Raglione and next door to Dr. Paul "Edward" Zuelke who had married the red-haired Inarose who had been stranded in the shower and then later caught on fire. Dr. Zuelke had also delivered three of Dee and Ed's four children. Dee initially felt slightly uncomfortable, living so close to these doctors, transported back to a time when she was instructed to address reverently any doctor as "sir." That soon faded, as both doctors were her friends and treated her as an equal.

The large boisterous 2 North group enjoyed having loud, raucous parties at Dee and Ed's. Their house became the unofficial St. Vincent's annex, even hosting people when it snowed so more staff could get to work. One doctor later remembered his days as an intern when he was summoned to one of these parties, jokingly referring it to as "hazing" of the younger set.

The 2 North crew would often reminisce about their days at the old hospital.

"Remember that patient in 236, bed 4?" they would laugh. "Remember the man with the hernia in Room 240, bed 2?" they'd remark. No one outside of the group had any idea who or what they were talking about. One had to marvel that they could remember not only every patient and their affliction, but also the room and bed number. Yet at the same time, it was as if a golden era of medicine had slipped by.

For a few years, the old hospital sat crumbling on its 12.5

acres, with peeling plaster, heaps of rubble and broken windows. *The Oregonian* newspaper summed it up:

> "The ghosts of the 1.1 million people who lived and died at the 80-year-old hospital were now silent. Gone were the cries of the 75,000 babies who had been brought into the world there; the Peter Pan wallpaper now torn and faded in the nursery. Above the now abandoned admissions desk, a painted cross sat with the words, 'Believe me, when you did it to one of the least of my brethren here, you did it to me.'"

The old hospital's price tag was $1 million and included the 11 magnificent huge stained-glass windows in the old chapel of the hospital. An ad in the newspaper with the headline, "Biggest Salvage Sale Yet!" promoted doors, sinks, toilets and more for sale. The stair posts of 2 North were one of the last things to be salvaged. They were bought by some of Ozzy's Girls and re-sold at the new hospital's gift shop. Alumnae and staff also bought other furniture, meticulously going through the old Nurses' Home for treasures. Rags was one of the salvagers, carefully picking through the rubble to find a stair post, railing and the ultimate find, the door to 2 North. He repurposed it all as a bar in his basement, proudly displaying the beautifully salvaged material.

After vandals looted the crumbling building, it was finally sold. The company that bought it said if they used dynamite, it would take two seconds to destroy it. They chose instead to sell the two million bricks at 18 cents apiece; the rest was taken to the dump. After it fell to a wrecking ball in 1977, a single boiler stack stubbornly remained. The demolition company tried three times to demolish it with explosives, with the final round successful in December 1977. It was as if Mother Joseph herself was watching with a sly smirk. Eventually, luxury condominiums were built on the hospital's sacred ground.

Peter Grant, *Oregon Journal* staff writer, chronicled it on August 2, 1977:

> "With a bit of imagination, it is possible to observe the perspective St. Vincent Hospital had on Portland's history. A squint of the eyes and the peeling paint becomes the hopeful faces of victims of influenza epidemics of post-World War I, the Great Depression years and the Columbus Day storm."

Dee once tried to capture the feeling of the old hospital by writing about it as well:

> "Even though the old red brick building of Portland's St. Vincent Hospital is now demolished, if you listen closely, you will hear the soft tread of nurses' footsteps on the white tiled floors of those long hallways and perhaps the jingle of the sisters' rosary beads and keys."

Sister Mary Laureen stepped down soon after the move with hushed whispers about the need to professionalize the role of administrator. She had been the first woman administrator of a hospital in the Portland area, named as one of the "Women of Accomplishment" in 1970 by the local newspaper. In the true spirit of Mother Joseph and Mother Mary Theresa, Sister Mary Laureen had accomplished more with her quiet dignity than most could dream in a lifetime.

When the first layperson, Thomas J. Underriner, became administrator, the Sisters of Providence's nearly 100-year reign firmly came to an end. The sisters were still involved, tending to the sick, but medicine's quickly developing pace and the hospital's growth and future plans continued without them in charge. The hospital's plans were altered as time went by, but the long-promised medical office buildings and parking structures were eventually built. Sister Mary Laureen laughed at the latter, remembering how they had set the hospital back from the road so that the patients would have a view. Now, the view on the lower floors of the hospital featured the parking structures.

Sister Mary Laureen would continue her spiritual care work in the Providence system. But first, Sister had a debt to pay: Dr. Raglione's years of volunteer work needed to be rewarded somehow.

Sister Mary Laureen soon made good on that debt: She found herself caring for Rags and Joan's seven children, ranging in age from 5 to 18, while the couple went on a five-week trip to Italy with Jim and Ann Blickle. Though she was now a renowned pioneer administrator, Sister Mary Laureen wasn't too savvy in the kitchen and the teenagers pushed her limits, while the youngest, Mary, needed lots of attention. Sister Mary Laureen, a "Woman of Accomplishment," meekly drove the kids in a carpool and wondering if this trade-off had been a fair one. She must have decided that it was; years later at her 100th birthday celebration, she referred to the Ragliones as a "branch of my family."

THE LEGACY OF OZZY'S GIRLS

The bond of Ozzy's Girls lived on after the closure of the St. Vincent School of Nursing—if only in the graduates' memories. Fortunately, in 1912, St. Vincent graduates had the forethought to organize themselves into an alumnae association. Their first member was the school's initial graduate, Rose Philpot, and a rapidly growing group soon followed. The St. Vincent Nurses Alumnae Association met every year from 1912 on, fittingly on the Feast of St. Vincent—the sacred July 19.

The alumnae continued with this tradition over the years, now calling it "Homecoming," and the reunions starting getting more elaborate, evolving into day-long events. During the 1940s, Ozzy was president of the Alumnae Association, hosting special events during the day, such as honoring those nurses who were serving in the Army Corps. After these ceremonies, all the graduates would gather for a formal luncheon.

Eventually, Homecoming became an evening banquet. The alumnae began inviting doctors who had been influential in their lives, as well as administrators from the hospital and university. Certain classes were honored if it was their big anniversary—25th, 30th, 40th, 50th, and even 60th. The women came from all over the country, many of them getting together for lunch or a post-Homecoming party with just their classmates. The children of many Ozzy's Girls soon learned nothing—*absolutely nothing*—could interfere with the crucial day: July 19.

The St. Vincent Nurses Alumnae Association eventually became an official nonprofit, with written bylaws and a board of directors. In fact, Dee acted as president and later treasurer for several years. At Homecoming, she was designated as the mistress of ceremonies, presiding over the event, trying to keep the gathering lively and meaningful. Many of Ozzy's Girls would come early, bustling through the halls to volunteer for the event, setting up decorations or checking others in. Chaos would soon ensue with Dee and Dorothy in charge and laughingly arguing over minor details.

Sister Mary Laureen, who now went by her birth name Rita, always made sure she attended. With her now short white curls, she was assigned to say the opening prayer and light the candle for those friends who were watching from heaven.

Ozzy was there, too, of course. She would never have missed it. Still walking ramrod straight, she had now beautiful white hair, softly curling about her face, her eyebrows still black and her eyes alight with laughter behind big glasses.

Ozzy had her fair share of sadness, though. After her mother died, she traveled to Hawaii in 1965, where she accidentally ran into Ross Jeckell, a former classmate from the Yukon. They married in 1969 at the age of 62. Unfortunately, he only lived two years following their marriage. It was a fairy tale, she once said in a rare moment of sentimentality.

Ozzy had no children—her surrogate children were her former students. They proclaimed themselves "her girls," even as they aged. Throughout the years, many of the alumnae traveled out to Ozzy's rambling house or over to Dee's house to reminisce about their days together. They had parties where they performed skits filled with inside jokes. Georgina Crater, who had commanded the emergency room at the old hospital, was the treasurer for decades and held the purse strings tight for the alumnae board, never wanting them to spend a penny. A short woman with a gray bun, she wore a permanent pursed-lip expression that didn't match her light heart, especially when she played the banjo. When she picked away at the instrument, the group danced and laughed. They continued sharing all the same inside jokes— even though they were graduates from various years.

As time passed, the alumnae realized their legacy had to be broader than just them and their memories. The women knew they needed to find a way to continue to help others. That solution soon came about.

The Homecoming on July 19, 1971, was a hot day in Portland. The room got even warmer when Alumnae President Evelyn Connor took the microphone and announced the organization of the Harriett E. Osborn Jeckell Foundation to Ozzy's complete surprise. The foundation would be started with a generous $3,000 gift. With whimsical humor, Dr. Shields passed a large sombrero around the room, raising $327 in additional funds. Ozzy's smile lit up the room, even if she protested just a little. The HEOJ Fund became a firmly established nonprofit.

For a time, the HEOJ Fund also funded two annual educational seminars for nurses at St. Vincent Hospital. Ongoing education was important to Ozzy, and therefore, this aspect was also a priority for the alumnae. Ozzy was able to see the breadth of her legacy fulfilled, even attending some of the seminars.

Georgina Crater's frugality paid off, and in 1989, the small group had a sizeable amount to donate. Others donated as well, eventually raising hundreds of thousands of dollars in the name of the woman who they said was a teacher, motivator, disciplinarian and a friend to all "her girls." The endowment fund honored Ozzy's legacy of her desire for all nurses to be highly educated. The alumnae achieved their goal; to this day, the HEOJ Fund provides several nursing scholarships at the University of Portland. For many years, Dee and Dorothy went out to meet the scholarship recipients at the University of Portland's annual Scholarship Reception. They would smile on the way, loving the opportunity to meet these young University of Portland nursing students (now both men and women). They would laugh about how different the students' training would be from their own.

Ozzy was given even more honors over the years, including the University of Portland's medal for outstanding service to the community. The university even commissioned a portrait by a local artist of Ozzy to be hung in the education complex.

The St. Vincent Nurses Alumnae and their annual Homecomings continued. They eventually raised money for a plaque for Sister Genevieve, who ran the school from 1925 to 1944. The alumnae were anxious that her legacy would not be forgotten. The plaque was given to the University of Portland to be hung in the College of Nursing.

The group established an Alumnae of the Year award in 1938; Dee was honored with it in 1988. Dorothy Kennedy was chosen to present it to her and said the following about Dee in her tribute:

"During her nursing career, she has been dedicated to the highest standards and principles of caring for patients in all aspects of their needs. She has always been an example to those with whom she has worked, teaching them as well as working with them side by side. I think it would be fair to say that patient contact was and still is her first love of nursing...She has the respect of those whom she supervises as well as her coworkers and is held in the highest esteem by the medical staff not only for her professional judgment, but for her nursing knowledge and skills...Many of you have worked with her and would agree that she has always given of herself to the profession. Her personality is always shining and of a positive nature."

Dee only smiled, looking downward at her folded hands. However, afterwards the award's gold medallion necklace, engraved with STV on the front, could always be seen around Dee's neck.

A few years later, in 1991, Harriett Osborn Jeckell died of a cerebral hemorrhage at the age of 85. She was a true nurse whose compassion and respect for humankind was legendary. When asked about the hardships of nursing, she once scoffed. "I never thought such a thing," she said, straightening her erect spine. "I don't think I was really that great. But my nurses think so, so I guess I must have spread something good somewhere."

Ozzy's Girls continued with their Homecomings, now walking past a portrait of Ozzy as they entered the banquet. The Alumnae Association was catered to by the CEO of the hospital at the time, Janice Burger, as well as Carolyn Winter and Kevin Finn of the Development Office. The alumnae were a tough group; the board often met with the hospital administrators to ensure their fund was secure and their plans for Homecoming went on without a hitch. They of course still penciled in July 19 as a sacred day.

In 2012, the St. Vincent Nurses Alumnae Association celebrated their 100th Homecoming Reunion. Word soon spread about this very special Homecoming, and a young doctor from a completely different generation learned about Ozzy's Girls. Though he had never worked with any of them, he greatly admired this group of resilient women and offered to buy engraved champagne glasses for a special toast. This thoughtful man wanted his gesture to be anonymous. Dee thought back to that champagne toast the night before graduation. With misty eyes, she agreed it was a perfect idea. She ordered a few hundred champagne glasses engraved with STV and the group raised them in honor of themselves and all those who had tread the stairs of old St. Theresa Hall.

Dee's toast was simple: "To those nurses who came before us, to our old friends who couldn't be here today, to the physicians and friends who have supported us throughout the years, to the nuns, professors, and doctors that taught us, and to us—those present today. Finally, to the anonymous donor who generously provided these glasses of champagne. Cheers!"

Dr. Ugo Raglione was among the doctors who stood to honor the nurses who he said had a great deal of influence over physicians. Retired now, his black hair mostly gray, he still wore his big glasses and lazy wide smile. "You helped convert medical students full of knowledge into doctors," drawled Rags. "I was one of them." His wife, Joan, Class of 1952, sat by his side and simply smiled knowingly.

Janice Burger, Providence St. Vincent's CEO, was there as well. "Every July 19 when we celebrate your graduations, I see what family you are," she remarked.

Among those honored that night was Barbara Benson Sharkey, a graduate of the Class of 1931, celebrating an incredible 81st anniversary. She had spent a lifetime as one of Ozzy's Girls and couldn't have been prouder.

The reunions continued over the next few years, the attendees' hair getting whiter, their health declining. Years of lifting patients with no mechanical beds, and the other physical labor they all had performed throughout the years, had taken its toll. They suffered aching backs and arthritic hips. Despite their health, they still continued to come, even if it meant wheeling in their oxygen tanks.

Isabel Booth, from the Cadet Class of 1947 and a member of the board, manned the famous spiked punch every year. She watched the incoming ladies and with a grin, asked her good friend Dee slyly: "Where's the walker parking?"

Homecoming was now held in the St. Vincent Medical Office Building, east of the main hospital. The ladies filed in, past the large picture of Ozzy, receiving corsages from Susie Matlock, an administrative assistant at the hospital, who had become the official florist of the St. Vincent Nurses Alumnae. Now children and even some grandchildren escorted their loved ones. The ladies posed for class photos and pored over displayed scrapbooks. The University of Portland recipients of the HEOJ Fund also attended. Wide-eyed and wondering what in the world they had stumbled into, the students left with a new admiration for this amazing group of ladies who shared such vibrant memories. As the women talked, it was as if they were magically transported back to their time at the school.

In 2016, the dwindling group of Ozzy's Girls sat down to make an important decision: Should they retire their annual celebration in glory or keep their reunions going? After 104 years, they decided it was time, and if they were going to go out, they'd go out strong.

At the last Homecoming, as many graduates who were physically able made the trip. It was a festive affair. Dee's granddaughter Delanie and her friend modeled old nurses' uniforms—one in a pin-striped version from the 1920s and another wearing Dee's from the 1940s. As they walked to the East Wing, current medical personnel simply stopped in their tracks and stared, wondering if the girls had been beamed in from a different era. The girls stood at the entrance in their blue capes with red lining and the STV on the collars, greeting all the guests. Many of the alumnae stopped just to stroke the uniform with their frail hands, smiling with watery eyes. In true Ozzy fashion, however, many of the alumnae inspected the girls twice over, commenting that their shoes were certainly not regulation and no jewelry would have been allowed.

The alumnae raised their glasses in one last toast to themselves, those who had come before them and finally, to Dee, who was credited with keeping Homecoming going, as well as visiting the sick alumnae throughout the years. Mostly, they were just happy that the memories of what they had endured and shared were kept alive.

Ozzy's Girls shared memories each year at Homecoming, but they also liked to write about their experiences in their biannual newsletter, the *Vincenette*, written and edited over the years by Dorothy and Dee and later just Dee, with the help of her daughters. The alumnae often cited their years in training as the greatest time in their lives.

Why did they keep Homecoming going for so long? Dee answered that readily in the *Vincenette*:

"For those of us who are graduates from St. Vincent Hospital School of Nursing and the University of Portland, there is a feeling of closeness to our classmates and other fellow alumnae. Our commitment made us a very special group, caring and concerned for each other. Our organization is a unique and outstanding one, of which we all can be proud. We kept the hospital running during the war years. We lived together, we ate together, we prayed together."

One graduate's daughter felt compelled to write to Dee, after reading her words:

"Mom's greatest accomplishment was graduating from St. Vincent School of Nursing. Her training there permeated throughout her life."

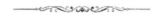

As Ozzy's Girls left that night in 2016, they drove past the sign that now said "Providence St. Vincent Medical Center"—a name they secretly smirked at, noting quietly it would always just be St. Vincent Hospital to them.

The massive building was a far cry from the one where they had trained. St. Vincent had now become a thriving medical center, later adding two more buildings, one aptly named Mother Joseph Plaza. Its doctors, nurses and staff members hurry down the halls on their way to help patients, walking sometimes obliviously past black-and-white photos of Mother Joseph and Mother Mary Theresa. In a case further down the hall, there are photos of Ozzy's Girls, smiling with their blue capes and white gloves. A campus garden, the Sister Rita Peace Garden, which was added in 2018 on Sister Rita's 100th birthday, remains as a silent, living legacy to a true pioneer. In the corner of the east building there is a photo of Rags with his construction hat on, a small plaque in his honor. The images, gardens, and other tributes are blurred into the landscape—a time mostly forgotten.

Someone once said St. Vincent Hospital's foundation was built on the backs of Ozzy's Girls and nuns, especially those who kept the hospital going during times of trial, with no money and the challenge of very little modern medicine. Their presence is still felt if you stop and savor their spirit, which graces the halls and most importantly the soul of caregiving.

ONCE A NURSE, ALWAYS A NURSE

And what happened in Dee's nursing career? In the 1970s, Dee enjoyed her days on 7 East, but her time there didn't last. She was soon tapped to join the hospital's administration. Torn between directly providing patient care or moving into administration where she might affect long-term change, she chose the latter. Dee became the associate director of surgical nursing services in the mid-1970s around the age of 50.

In this new role, Dee was also assigned to help fundraise to finish the ninth floor of the hospital. The plan was for the ninth floor to be a much-needed cancer unit. Dee was the nurse's representative on a board full of prominent Portland business executives. She felt a little out of her depth, but held her own as usual, advocating for the need for this floor. As a symbolic gesture to kick off the fundraising drive, Dee was chosen to throw up a basketball between two Trail Blazers, the city's NBA Team that had recently won the national championship. Flanked on either side by Trail Blazers Geoff Petrie and Bob Gross, the 5-foot-2 Dee looked even tinier, beaming with her nurse's cap, giving her a few more inches in height. The press loved it, and the photo attracted a lot of attention. Eventually, the ninth floor was finished and included a plaque with her name and the other members of the committee.

In 1982, Dee was promoted to associate director of critical care nursing. Around the same time, her old friend Dorothy Kennedy was also promoted to be her counterpart—only on the medical side of the house. The old days of Dee and Dorothy running around 2 North all day were now mirrored, only it was the entire hospital. Dee would wave to Dorothy, now both answering constant pages, as they both flew down the hallways in different directions. Dee would often take the back stairs to more quickly navigate the vast hospital, running from one emergency to another. In fact, one doctor once remarked when he first came to St. Vincent Hospital, he heard the constant "Dee Wallo to..." over the hospital's loudspeaker. "Who is this woman who seemingly needs to be in every place at every moment?" he wondered.

Technology finally caught up with Dee, though, and she grudgingly consented to having a pager affixed to her new uniform, which consisted of plain clothes and a white lab coat. She gave up the uniform, but still jiggling in her pockets were her surgical scissors, tape and of course, forceps—a valued tool she often said she could use to fix anything. Though responsible for all surgical wards, operating rooms, the recovery room, intensive care and the emergency room, Dee could often be found in a patient's room, assessing him or her. On her desk was a continual pile of paperwork that she did not want to deal with. She'd much rather be in a patient's room or chatting with the nurses under her supervision.

In addition to the daily work of managing surgical areas, Dee focused her efforts on building the intensive care unit and later on creating a cardiac recovery unit. She told anyone who would listen about the need to expand care for critical patients. Dee traveled to look at advancing medical machinery, marveling at the technology. She couldn't wait to buy it and save more lives.

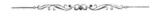

DESPITE HER MISGIVINGS ABOUT DEE'S CAREER, DEE'S mother Theresa learned to lean on her daughter's knowledge and skill. Dee had become the nurse for the entire extended family. She was called constantly by family members for advice or requests to go with them to doctor's appointments. This weighed heavily on Dee, who was concerned about the power they were placing in her hands to help them make medical decisions. It also deeply affected her when someone she loved was hospitalized. She often was by a loved one's bedside, holding their hand when they passed, feeling the enormity of it all on her shoulders.

Dee was great at taking care of everyone, but sometimes she forgot to take care of herself. A typical nurse, she did not make a good patient.

In September 1984, shortly following her 60th birthday, Dee was home sick, suffering from what she thought was a stomach virus. Suddenly, she was in terrific pain and told Ed to take her to the hospital. Strong as always, he rolled her in a blanket and carried her into the Emergency Room. Her children, now grown, rushed to the hospital as well. The news wasn't good: Rags and Dr. Inahara agreed to operate, but they warned the family she might not survive the surgery—they surmised it was a grave bowel obstruction. Later that night as Dee's family sat in the empty, darkened hospital lobby, they looked up to see Rags and Dr. Inahara, still in their scrubs, walking toward them from the shadows, smiling and slapping each other on the back.

"That stupid Wallo," said Rags, never mincing words in his long, drawn-out drawl. "She let her appendix burst." They laughed mostly in relief that their old friend would be fine. The two would never let her forget it, and they took great joy in ribbing her later. Dee recovered on her beloved 7 East—the line became so long outside her room, her friend Joan Currie finally placed a guest book in the hall in lieu of visitors. Dee returned to work and continued her efforts to build the hospital's critical areas, especially in the areas of cardiac recovery.

Soon after, though, Rags ended up operating on his old friend again, but this time, it was just to repair a hernia. Rags fixed Dee up and she resided in her 7 East again, happy to catch up with her old friends. At the same time, she was worried about her oldest daughter MaryJo who was also in the hospital after having a minor procedure.

Dee was a mother first, a nurse second and of course, third, a terrible patient. Putting on a hospital robe, she wheeled her IV pole out of her hospital room doorway. Looking both ways, she casually strolled down the hall, as if taking a small walk. Taking one last look around, Dee darted for the service elevators, descending a couple floors.

Dee's daughter was resting quietly, only to look up and see her mother stroll in with her IV pole trailing behind her. Dee looked her daughter over and saw that she was recovering satisfactorily. Dee began to laugh, a hoarse, gasping sound, clutching her incision. She was obviously pleased at her cunning escape. Laughingly, she turned to slip quietly back upstairs before anyone was the wiser.

<hr />

IN 1985, ED RETIRED FROM THE POLICE BUREAU, AFTER rising to the rank of lieutenant. Dee desperately wanted to join him, but she wanted to wait until the new cardiac recovery unit she helped plan was built. So it wasn't until March 1987 that Dee retired at the age of 62—leaving after 40 years at St. Vincent.

The Oregonian reported later that a large crowd of friends and coworkers gathered on February 27 of that year to celebrate Dee's nursing career and wish her well in retirement. She received the "Vinnie," a statuette which honored distinguished service at St. Vincent. The Vinnie sat next to the Heritage Award she had already received in 1985 from the University of Portland.

"Compassion is a word everyone uses to describe Dee," said Wally Hathaway, RN, at the time to *The Oregonian*. "She personifies sensitivity."

Georgina Crater was there, minus the banjo. Never one to offer praise unless it was earned, she told *The Oregonian*: "She [Dee] has the kind of love feelings that nurses should have for people."

Jane Smith, assistant administrator for patient-care services agreed. "She is a strong leader, fair and loaded with common sense. She is very knowledgeable and treats all people with respect—whether they be housekeepers, administrators or doctors. Her constant goal is the best patient care possible. Roll all those traits into one person and you have Wallo."

"She would take us aside and tell us what we did wrong without making us feel bad about it," said Pat Van Loo, who worked on 2 North and later 7 East under Dee. "She'd just sidle up to us with a big smile and chat with us privately. She wanted us to be as successful as we could be."

Other praised Dee's patience, fairness, wisdom, sense of humor and "phenomenal stamina."

Perhaps the highest praise—or at least what meant the most to Dee—was the words from Ozzy herself, who seemed to have forgotten for the moment how many times she took Dee's cap away during training:

"I hired her when she first went to work at the hospital. She had been an excellent student when in training... She loved bedside nursing. She could solve problems and do the right thing."

Dee told *The Oregonian*:
"If I have been effective, it is because I have always liked what I was doing. I like people, and I generally enjoy caring for them. And I believe I must have a natural empathy and sympathy for patients and their families. I have never been unhappy in my career....

"Many people have been right alongside of me, working arm-in-arm and hand-in-hand. I don't think I've done anything exceptional. Just try to work hard. I enjoyed patient care, patient contact. That's really what it's all about. Those years down in 2 North at the old hospital were very exciting times because of the advances that were going on in medicine and because of patient satisfaction—being a part of that. The hospital will always be a part of me. From where I live, I can see the hospital. I stand on my deck and say, 'There it is.'"

"It's two different worlds," Dee said of the old hospital and new one. "I think I had the best of all of it."

Dee dreamed of a retirement filled with travel and fun with Ed, but it wasn't to be. Dee saw changes in her husband now that she was home with him during the day. Soon, he was diagnosed with pugilistic dementia. In current day, it undoubtedly would be diagnosed as Chronic Traumatic

Encephalopathy (CTE), a neurodegenerative disease caused by repeated head injuries (from his boxing days). A short two years later, Dee was forced to place him in a care facility—the most difficult decision of her life. Though she had cared for countless people over the years, she was unable to care for her still physically strong husband and it broke her heart. Though Ed's memory faded regarding most people, he still always recognized the love of his life, lighting up when Dee walked in his care facility every day.

Dee was a fixture there, often feeding those in the dining room who couldn't feed themselves. As a seasoned caregiver, she readily tended to the patients' needs so much so that visitors often mistook her for an employee and asked her to do extra work for their loved one.

One day, as she traveled through the dining room, Dee came upon a man slumped in his wheelchair. After a quick pulse check, she calmly said, "I think this one isn't going to eat his lunch." The horrified staff quickly scrambled to remove him. Dee was ever compassionate, but also had a bit of her mother's practicality.

Still, when Ed died in 1996 with Dee holding his hand, it hit her hard. She carried on, though, soldiering through life as always, volunteering and taking care of her grandchildren (she would eventually have nine). She loved life, enjoyed being active and traveling with Dorothy, as well as other trips with Ann Clark and Schmidty.

Dee embraced this new life, despite her longing for Ed. Faith continued to be an important part of her life and she lived it. She visited her mother, Theresa, now in a nursing home (her father, Frank, had passed several years earlier at the age of 95) as well as her Uncle Tony. When both passed away, she continued volunteering at the church, making sandwiches for those less fortunate and counting the offering after mass. She also volunteered at Theresa's former nursing home, wheeling in the residents for a Sunday afternoon of bingo. She cheated on their behalf, always wanting everyone to feel like a winner. Dee taught some of her grandkids how to drive and she never missed a sporting event, play or school activity.

She had no idea that her life was once again going to take a slight turn.

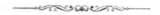

"OH MY GOD, IT'S DEE WALLO!" DR. SHARFF EXCLAIMED.

Dee felt like she was dreaming. She was back on the floor again, running to a code in the emergency room. She heard Dr. Jeffrey Sharff's voice. She went back to sleep, wondering why she was back at work if she had retired.

Later, Dee woke up and instantly knew she was in the intensive care unit. She looked at her nurse, recognizing her as someone she had worked with. Trying to speak, she realized quickly she had an intubation tube in, connected to a ventilator to help her breathe. She glanced to her left and met her daughter Terri's worried eyes. She gave Terri a fierce look in return, her brown eyes snapping, silently reminding her that she had often told her no extraordinary measures should be done if it came to that.

"The tube is only short term, Mom," Terri started to explain, and Dee's eyebrows raised as if to say, "It better be." The doctor came in soon after, extubating her, gently pulling the tube out, and Dee reached her small hand toward Terri.

"Swanson," she rasped out, her voice thin from the intubation. Terri looked at the nurse helplessly. "I don't understand," she said.

"Swanson," whispered Dee again emphatically.

The nurse smiled. "I thinking she's asking for Dr. Jeff Swanson," she explained. Dee nodded vigorously. The family soon learned that Dr. Swanson had come to St. Vincent as an intern and had been long schooled by Dee, even coming over to the house for the usual parties. He was now a prominent cardiothoracic surgeon, and Dee knew she needed him when she woke up in the ICU.

One of Dee's physician friends explained later that it wasn't just because she was weak that she had fallen when she entered the emergency department that early morning. It also was not an asthma attack. In fact, her heart had simply stopped as soon as she walked in.

"You left it too long, Dee," he told her on his visit, shaking his head. "If you were across the street, we couldn't have saved you."

Another doctor took a more positive approach, bowing to divine intervention: "What kind of amazing life have you led that when your heart stopped, it would be in one of the premier cardiac centers in the country?"

Soon, many of Dee's other physician friends descended upon her: Dr. Raglione and Dr. Inahara led the pack as well as Dr. Donald Sutherland, her beloved cardiologist who had taken care of her for years since her heart failure in the 1960s. He had just retired and her new cardiologist, Dr. Craig Walsh, accompanied him. Additional doctors came, all from her days as a nurse. They came to be reunited, but also to stand in solidarity because they knew convincing Dee to finally have cardiac surgery was going to take a major intervention. They were all secretly a little frightened at the thought of her reaction.

"It's time to get the valve done," they said collectively, crowding into her room. Knowing they were right, Dee grudgingly agreed. She had always been told she had rheumatic fever as a child, and a valve damaged by that infection is usually irreparable. Thus, she would need a new valve to repair her heart. She had witnessed those early valve surgeries in the 1960s, and though they were groundbreaking, they were also high-risk with a long recovery. Dee had seen too much over the years. She maintained she wouldn't do it until they invented a valve that she could literally just swallow. Unfortunately, medicine had advanced, but not quite that far.

Dr. Swanson arrived on the scene following the intervention with Dee. "Who the hell is Rose?" he barked with a glint in his eye as he walked in holding her chart. Dee laughed, knowing no one knew her real name. Dr. Swanson agreed to do the surgery later that week on Good Friday. Dee frowned at the timing.

"What if I just go home for Easter with my family and I'll come right back on the following Monday?" she bargained. Dr. Swanson simply shook his head no.

When Dr. Swanson came out of surgery on that fateful Good Friday to talk to Dee's anxious family, he smiled. She apparently did not have rheumatic fever as a child, he explained. She probably had suffered just a serious infection that had damaged her valve. The valve was fixable, and he had repaired it. He jokingly told her he gave her a 20-year warranty on his work.

The weekend following her surgery was Easter Weekend, and the hospital was quiet. Dee's family gathered outside of cardiac recovery, staring at the poster of Dr. Swanson in the lobby. They were incredibly grateful, but becoming increasingly worried as they watched other patients who had surgeries after Dee get transferred to the cardiac floor of the hospital.

By Monday, Dee's daughters became frantic. When Dr. Sutherland walked by, they grabbed him by the arm, asking him why Dee was still in cardiac recovery. Was there something they didn't know, they asked. Was she not improving?

Dr. Sutherland was compassionate and promised an answer. He soon returned with Dr. Walsh, who reassured the daughters. He told them the cardiac recovery nurses knew

Dee, or knew of her, and they were reluctant to let her go to the floor. The nurses wanted to continue to oversee her care, and he would probably need to wrestle her away from their grip eventually, knowing others needed the specialized unit more than her.

Her daughters then took a deep breath, knowing she was improving. Life would go on. And it did.

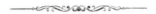

IN THE YEARS THAT FOLLOWED, DEE HAD A FEW HEALTH issues and was hospitalized from time to time. She watched when the nurses came in, sometimes going to the computer first rather than to speak with her or even greet her. Since she had no poker face to speak of, her face instantly read annoyance that documenting everything had become the priority rather than the patient. It was a sign of the times, and she understood the legal pressures the medical field was under and how technology helped the communication flow between doctors, nurses and departments. She never blamed the nurses and always encouraged them. She continued to recognize exceptional health care, even once reassuring a nervous IV nurse who was told Dee was a "legend." "It's okay. You're doing fine," Dee said, patting the nurse's hand.

Dee's doctor who was in charge of ensuring that her heart stayed in rhythm was Dr. Tony Garvey. She often saw Dr. Garvey, lobbing rapid-fire questions in his direction about her care. Dr. Garvey insisted he treated her and made decisions just like he would for his own mother.

"But do you like your mother?" retorted Dee, her brown eyes glinting, her eyebrows wickedly wiggling.

Dee was still active in helping the University of Portland's School of Nursing, and she was asked if she would act as a mentor for students. Readily agreeing, she hosted nursing students who came to her each semester. Dee said she tried to not to bore them with history, but impart her passion for patient care instead, hoping to affect change one student at a time.

One family friend who was studying to be a physician's assistant loved hearing Dee's stories. Touched, Dee gave her an old textbook. The student brought it into one of her classes and her fellow students coveted it, thumbing through it and discovering the medical terms of the 1940s.

Dr. Swanson's skill gave Dee another 12 years. She was able to watch her grandchildren grow up, with the youngest two turning 16. She was active until the last year, when she began to slow down. Unfortunately, the last two months of pneumonia and a fractured hip put her in and out of the hospital and in the same nursing home where she had helped the patients cheat at bingo. She smiled through the pain; her eyes still bright.

Dr. Raglione came to visit her. Now a widower, his beloved Joan had passed three years prior. Dee and Rags joked about getting old, but couldn't stop smiling at each other. Neither had to voice the connection they shared.

Dee talked a lot about her time in New Jersey during those days, reliving the time with Ed where there had been no children, just the two of them. Her eyes misted, telling those stories from so long ago, their memories so vivid.

One night as Dee's blood pressure dropped dangerously low, the decision was made to move her to ICU. "I under-stand she's precious to this hospital," said the hospitalist, who had only just met her. "We'll take the best care of her."

The family soon learned that she would not be waking up —that all measures that she would want had been exhausted. Janice Burger, then the CEO of the hospital, kindly visited Dee's family to ensure they had what they needed.

Dee's family took turns visiting her in ICU. They covered

her with a quilt the hospital gave them and made a playlist of her favorite songs that played continuously. The ICU nurses quietly did their jobs, competent and caring. Dee's children wished they could tell their mom how much she would approve of the ICU nurses' care.

Dee's children and grandchildren prayed with the hospital chaplain, Father Chris, and their family priest, Monsignor Tim Murphy. They walked around outside and wandered the halls, lost in thought. They often went up to the second floor, where a giant tribute wall had been hung in Dee's honor. Just seeing her smiling face brought her closer.

They looked at the other photos of Dee's nursing friends, Dr. Raglione, Sister Rita, Ozzy and the many other people they had grown up around, hearing stories about the hospital. They realized they were surrounded by Dee's legacy, not in just the ICU or cardiac recovery, and the walls of her beloved hospital, but with them and their children who camped out at the hospital, and whose hearts were breaking.

Early on in the ICU, Dee simply said, "Ed," while holding her granddaughter's hand. Later the next night, she died peacefully in the place she had built. She was undoubtedly in Ed's arms within seconds. "Fly Me to the Moon" was playing.

The tribute wall still hangs in her honor near the Nursing Service offices on the second floor of the main hospital and is in a hallway near the cardiac operating rooms. Next to her photo it says:

As a graduate of the St. Vincent Hospital School of Nursing, Rose Marie "Dee" Wallo served most of her student years during a time of momentous change in nursing: World War II. Across the nation, nurses were called upon to care for wounded soldiers and for the first time, to make treatment decisions.

The St. Vincent nursing school participated in the U.S. Cadet Nurse Corps program, which subsidized the training of vitally needed nurses. Nurses emerged from the war years with specialty skills and with newfound stature as health care professionals.

Ms. Wallo witnessed the explosion of knowledge and medical technology that showered nurses with opportunities to learn, to innovate, and to become true partners in health care delivery. As a nursing leader, she worked with physicians to bring sophisticated treatments to St. Vincent Hospital. She made invaluable contributions to nursing education and the development of nursing care standards.

Throughout her career as staff nurse, supervisor, and associate nursing director, and in her leadership of the nursing school alumnae association, Dee Wallo stayed focused on bringing competent, caring nursing practice to patients. She taught and guided with wisdom, wonder and abundant joy.

It certainly captures Dee's impact, but maybe a patient's wife summed her up just as well in describing why patient care was so important. She wrote Dee on November 15, 1954, after the death of her husband and the note obviously meant something to Dee who kept it. Though it's written about Dee, it's a reminder of how much impact a nurse can have on a patient as well as a patient's loved ones.

"To all of us, you are a special person heaven sent... your light of compassion was precious. We will never forget your quick flash of smile and quick way of bringing out some little piece of good news when you could—nor your dark hair flying behind you as you sped about, your chosen wink. If all this seems very personal—and you hesitate—let it be read—you must remember that all the fine and wonderful patients who are in rare affliction, are your friends. Never let it be forgotten. Blessed be you for your countless deeds of kindness."

THE END

THANK YOU

Thanks for reading Ozzy's Girls.

For more stories, photos, video, memories and more, visit
ozzysgirls.com

To donate to Ed and Dee Scholarship Fund at the University
of Portland, visit edanddeewallo.com

NOTES

"Alumnae Honors War Nurses." *The Oregonian*, 20 July 1941.

Beadle, Roy. "St. Vincent's Hospital, 75 Years Old, Grew From Humble Start." *The Beacon*, 12 May 1950.

"Biggest Salvage Sale Yet." *The Oregonian*, n.d.

"Blickle, Chuck [Interview]." 2020.

"Bonjour." *The Oregonian*, 30 July 1978.

Budnick, Nick. "Famed Heart Surgeon Rejoins OHSU faculty" *The Oregonian* (unknown).

Centennial Observance, St. Vincent Hospital, St. Vincent Hospital, Portland, OR, 1975.

"Citation of the Week." *The Oregonian*, 31 Oct. 1943.

"Clark, Helen [Interview]." 2020.

"Class of 1954," Scrapbook.

Clyde, Velma. "Mother Joseph Recalled as Nuns Mark 100 Years of Hospital Service." 17 May 1975.

College of Nursing brochure, University of Portland, Portland, OR, 1950.

College of Nursing admissions brochure, University of Portland, Portland, OR, n.d.

"Coming Down." *The Oregonian*, 22 Nov. 1977.

Commencement Exercises, University of Portland, Portland, OR, 1950.

Cummins, Jean. "Nursing the First Fifty Years." *University of Portland: Portland Magazine*, 1985.

"Days Numbered for Old Hospital." *Oregon Journal*, 2 Aug. 1977.

"Dee Rennie Wallo, Private Collection."

Digital Collection, Providence, providencearchives.contentd-m.oclc.org/digital/collection/p15352coll5.

"Father John Hooyboer Obituary." *The Oregonian*, 1995.

Ferlic, Anne. "*Vincenette.*" 1970.

Ferschweiler, Rita. *The Crescent*, St. Vincent Hospital, 1971.

Ferschweiler, Rita. "*Vincenette.*" 2007.

"Foundation to Officer Nursing Education." *Catholic Sentinel*, 23 July 1971.

Garner, Julie. "Catholic Hospitals on Cutting Edge of Health Care throughout Oregon History." *Catholic Sentinel*, 16 Sept. 1984.

Goetzel, Ed. "Portland's Women of Accomplishment." *Oregon Journal*, 2 Feb. 1971.

Grant, Peter. "Days Numbered for Old Hospital." *Oregon Journal*, 2 Aug. 1977.

Guernsey, John. "40 Years of Caring Praised." *The Oregonian*, 26 Feb. 1987.

"Harriett Osborn Jeckell Obituary." *The Oregonian*, 21 Sept. 1991.

"History of Holy Cross." *History of Holy Cross | University of Portland*, www.up.edu/holycross/history/index.html.

"Hospital Administrator Is Native Oregonian." *Valley Times*, 4 Mar. 1971.

"Hospital Drive Boosted." *The Oregonian*, Accessed 14 Feb. 1954.

"Hospital Milestone." *Unknown*, 26 Jan. 1996.

"Hospital Stack Tough to Topple." *The Oregonian*, 11 Dec. 1977.

Inahara, Toshio. *A Nisei, Right Place, Right Time*. Toshio Inahara, M.D., 2015.

Kennedy, D. (1988). Dee Rennie Wallo, Alumnae of the Year Award [Speech].

"Kennedy, Dorothy" [Interview]. 2019.

"Liefeld, Mary" [Interview]. 2021.

Lucia, Ellis. *Cornerstone, The Formative Years of St. Vincent—Oregon's First Hospital*. St. Vincent Hospital Medical Foundation, 1975.

"McCloskey, MaryJo" [Interview]. 2019.

McCurtain, Bruce. *Coming Down*. Portland, OR, 2 Nov. 1977.

"Medal Winners." *The Oregonian*, 9 May 1977.

"*Mobile Model*: Providence St. Vincent" 1993.

"*Mobile Model*: Providence St. Vincent." 1995.

"*Mobile Model*, Providence St. Vincent." 1 July 1997.

"Money 'Speeded By Prayer' Helped Keep Early Creditor from Closing St. Vincent." 13 May 1975.

"Mother Joseph Recalled as Nuns Mark 100 Years of Hospital Service." *The Oregonian*, 17 May 1975.

Murphy, Joe. "Northwest Native Saw 112 Years Unfold." *The Oregonian*, 1998.

"New Hospital, New Life." *Catholic Sentinel*, 5 Feb. 1971.

"New Wing Work at St. Vincent's Due to Start Tuesday in Modernizing Job." *The Oregonian*, 11 Mar. 1956.

"Nursing School Alums Get Together for 100th." *The Oregonian*, 19 July 2012.

"Old St. Vincent Hospital Falls on West Hills." *Unknown*, Dec. 1977.

"Oregon Journal." *2 Hospitals Mark Anniversary*, 13 May 1975.

Our Providence Tradition, Providence Health & Services, n.d.

Pardieck, Betty. "Sister Flora Mary Follows Lord's Direction." *Burbank Daily Review*, 27 May 1968.

Perry, Douglas. "Sister Rita Ferschweiler, Pioneering Hospital Administrator Who Led Providence St. Vincent 'over the Hill,' Dies at 102." *Oregonlive*, 29 Apr. 2020, https://www.oregonlive.com/portland/2020/04/sister-rita-ferschweiler-pioneering-hospital-administrator-who-led-providence-st-vincent-over-the-hill-dies-at-102.html.

Portland Magazine, "University of Portland." Winter 2016.

"Portland's Women of Accomplishment." *Oregon Journal*, 2 Feb. 1971.

"Postwar Health Problem: Nursing Jobs Go Begging." *The Oregonian*, 8 Dec. 1948.

Providence Spirit: In the Beginning, Providence, Portland, OR, 1999.

"Providence St. Vincent Boasts Frontier Tradition." *Catholic Sentinel*, 23 Feb. 1996.

"Providence St. Vincent Celebrates 125 Years." *Catholic Sentinel*, 14 July 2000.

"Retired Nurse Never Stopped Caring." *Gresham Outlook*, 15 Nov. 1986.

"Retired Portland Physician Dies at 85." *The Oregonian*, 23 Aug. 1993.

Richards, Suzanne. "Administrator Plans Directs Hospital Move." *Oregon Journal*, 15 Feb. 1971.

"Rita Marie Ferschweiler, SP Obituary." *Seattle Times*, 25 Apr. 2020.

"Scherzinger, Rose" [Interview]. 2020.

Shields, Ambrose. *I Remember When*, Ambrose Shields, Portland, OR, 2009.

"Sisters of Providence Online Edition." https://sistersofprovidence.net/jubilee-2013/70-years-rita-ferschweiler-sp/

"Sister Rita Ferschweiler, SP Private Collection."

St. Vincent School of Nursing [Bylaws]. (n.d.).

St. Vincent Hospital Admissions Brochure, 1965.

St. Vincent School of Nursing Admissions Brochure, n.d.

St. Vincent School of Nursing [Banquet invitations, programs]. (n.d.).

St. Vincent School of Nursing [Graduation Program] 1931.

"St. Vincent Hospital Grows with the Community." *Valley Times*, 4 Mar. 1971.

"St. Vincent Hospital Moves Patients With Speed, Cheer." *The Oregonian*, 11 Feb. 1971.

"St. Vincent Medical Center Bares Plans." *The Oregonian*, 1 July 1970.

St. Vincent Medical Foundation, Tentative Master Plan, n.d.

St. Vincent Nurses Alumnae. *The Harriett Osborn Jeckell Education Fund*, 2004.

"St. Vincent School of Nursing Graduation Banquet Program." 1931.

"St. Vincent's Has Roots in Northwest." *Northwest Examiner*, 1 Nov. 2009.

"St. Vincent's Proud History Continues." *Catholic Sentinel*, 18 July 1997.

"Story of Marie Schmitz." Received by Joeine Wegerbauer Coons, 1980.

"Supply of Nurses Short in Area." *The Oregonian*, 19 Dec. 1952.

Terry, John. "Nursing the First...." *The Oregonian*, 16 July 2000, p. A21.

Terry, John. "Two Courageous, Unstoppable Women Build St. Vincent, a Hospital for All." *The Oregonian*, 16 July 2000.

The Beacon, "University of Portland" July 1977.
The Crescent, St. Vincent Hospital Internal Newsletter. *1964-1968.*

"The Sisters of Providence Celebrate 125 Years of Service in the West." *Catholic Sentinel*, 31 Dec. 1981.

"Two Hospitals Started 100 Years Ago." *The Oregonian*, 22 June 1975.

University of Portland Bulletin. *College of Nursing 1950-1951.*

University of Portland St Vincent Hospital School. *Nursing College Admissions Brochure*, n.d.

"Van Loo, Pat" [Interview]. 2021.

"Wallo, Dee" [Interview]. 1990-2018.

Wallo, Dee. "*Vincenette*." 1971.

"Wallo, Edward" [Interview]. 2019.

"Wallo, Steve" [Interview]. 2019.

Vincenette, 1980-2018

Vincentian, St. Vincent's Hospital newspaper. 1 Aug. 1931.

Vincentury, St. Vincent's Hospital newsletter, 1981.

Zuelke, Inarose. *Inarose Zuelke: Autobiography,* Portland, OR. n.d.

CPSIA information can be obtained
at www.ICGtesting.com
Printed in the USA
LVHW082320280921
698959LV00001B/1/J